MY OWN COURT

The Life Story

of

Tennis Legend

John Riggio

Mr. John A. Riggio

Dedication

To my daughter **_Nancy Xuwen Riggio_** for helping
me return to playing tennis.

Contents

Introduction

In the world of tennis, where dreams collide with reality, few players can claim a legacy as unique and multifaceted as that of John Anthony Riggio. This book is more than just a chronicle of my journey from a junior tennis hopeful to a distinguished professional player; it is a celebration of resilience, ingenuity, and the relentless pursuit of excellence in a sport defined by serious competition and playing sportsmanlike.

As one of the select few players to achieve victory in prestigious tournaments like the Eastern Tournament, the Manhattan Open, and the American Airlines Open, I lived both the highs of triumphant wins and the lows of fierce rivalries. My ground-breaking endeavors extend beyond the court—I was instrumental in the creation of a new pro tennis league designed specifically to ensure that players like myself could sustain a career while grappling with the ever-evolving landscape of professional sports.

This book delves into my singular experience of holding my own tennis court, both as a junior and an adult player—a rare feat that speaks volumes about my commitment and talent. Each chapter unpacks the vibrant tapestry of my career, including the incidents of breaking racquets in matches, a testament to my fierce tenacity and unyielding spirit during competition.

Behind every opportunity, there lay the crucial support of influential sponsors and a dedicated administrative coach whose belief in my potential propelled me forward. My journey was not just about climbing the ranks; it was about forging connections with top names in sports and society, gaining insights into their worlds while maintaining my personal integrity in the face of scandals and ethical issues that plagued the sport.

Yet, my story is also one of overcoming adversity. Faults in the ATP administrative office led to a chaotic and confusing array of names associated with my career. I had to navigate these complexities, changing my player name six times and enduring various misprints on tournament wins. This book addresses those challenges directly, aiming for clarity and unity under my rightful name—Mr. John Anthony Riggio.

My pathway to becoming a professional player was paved with self-initiative and determination. From creating my own tennis club in middle school and high school to picking up the phone and negotiating sponsorships, I navigated uncharted waters to keep my passion alive. I became a self-taught ambassador for the sport, educating my sponsors on how tournaments operated and implementing strategies that would help pave my way to the ATP.

In choosing to share my journey, I aim to inspire aspiring athletes, provide insights into the real workings of professional sports, and highlight the importance of perseverance and integrity. This book is not just my story but a testament to what can be achieved when passion meets purpose. Join me as we explore the ups and downs of a life dedicated to tennis—a journey where every swing of the racket, every changed name, and every hard-fought match converges into a narrative rich with lessons and triumphs. Welcome to the world of John Anthony Riggio, where the court is where it all happened.

Chapter One
The Origins of My Tennis Journey

Born Mr. John Anthony Riggio on September 26th, 1968 in Roslyn, NY, and raised in a Hamlet called Jericho, NY. This was located on Long Island, a suburb of New York City. My parents Mr. Michael Nicholas Riggio and Mrs. Rose Angela Ventimiglia liked this neighborhood because it was a new subdivision and a larger house than previously found. The area was positioned near the Long Island Railroad station at Hicksville, NY where my Father needed to commute to his job in Brooklyn, NY. He was employed by the Penn Railroad's print office. This was a good public service job and it encompassed working long hours.

My parents had previously lived in the Boroughs of Queens and Brooklyn in New York City. My father already had more of a long passage than my mother having been born in Passaic, New Jersey then moving to NYC were he was drafted into WWII in Europe. Afterwards, he lived for a number of years in Santa Barbara, California. Wounded but undeterred, he returned home to Brooklyn, NY to cultivate a new career for himself, trading construction for a long-term position with the Railroad. My mother was used to living in Brooklyn, NYC with a full time job with the Bell Phone company, she made frequent trips to her parents' summer home in Port Jefferson, NY.

My parents together with my two older brothers Paul and Philip and I formed a family unit united not just by blood, but by a shared ardor for tennis. In the warm embrace of my family's love, the seed of my passion for tennis was sown. It all began on sunlit afternoons at the local courts, where laughter mingled with the faint sound of racquets striking tennis balls.

I was just five years old, a small child fitted with a wooden racket that seemed almost too big for my tiny frame. My father was my first coach, a gentle yet firm guide, teaching me the basics of footwork, grip, and the thrill of competition. My mother, too, was right there beside us, her encouragement invaluable as she shared her own love for playing the game. I remember the excitement swelling in my chest as I first learned to hit the ball, the surprising crack of wood against fuzzy yellow felt echoing in my ears. However, it wasn't long before I tested the limits of my equipment. One fateful swing, full of youthful strength, resulted in the splintering of my wooden racket. The sound was sharp, a perfect metaphor for the revelation that would soon follow. My father, eyes wide with both astonishment and pride, took a moment to assess the scene before him. In just two minutes, he could see something within me — a spark, perhaps — that fueled his belief that I could become a professional tennis player.

Yet, even as he worked tirelessly, It was during these early years that tennis became our sanctuary. My father, Mr. Michael Riggio, shared his vision of success with me not as a mere fantasy but as a tangible possibility, rooted in his own experiences in the world of sports. He had been a dedicated tennis player, achieving the certified playing level of 4.5, and had a history steeped in competitive sports. He had the great will to win early in his life as a Boxer. Winning the championship bout at his High School in Brooklyn, NY.

Alongside my grandfather, Mr. Joseph Riggio, who grew to own a custom leather shoe business in a storefront located in Brooklyn, NY. Yet, it was Joseph's passion for sports business that truly set him apart from his peers.

Known for helping athletes navigate the treacherous waters of competition, he was licensed to sponsor tennis players and boxers alike. Together they visited the sporting events of the players they sponsored. Witnessing great professional sports playing and learning from the players' wins and losses.

Built from years of sports sponsoring experience my father said "You must always play honestly". This instilled a moral compass within me that would guide my decisions on and off the court. "The honest players are the ones who win in the long run. Sponsors need to know they can trust you." This lesson, one of integrity coupled with ambition, carved a niche within my heart, urging me to overcome the ordinary of life to seek greatness in my passion.

As I stood there, clutching the remnants of the broken racket, it became apparent that tennis was more than simply a sport; it was a gateway to understanding my family's rich tapestry of history and values. From a lineage that had traversed the Atlantic over a century ago — my great-grandfather escaping the limitations of a noble family in Catania, Italy, Europe — to establishing themselves in America with ambitions that blended tradition with opportunity, my family's journey was a testament to resilience and aspiration.

My mother's side of the family had a similar heritage and were from a noble family who lived outside of Palermo, Italy. They showed me photos and told stories of their estate where their ancestors raised horses for the Army as part of a service to their country. My grandmother Audenzia (Nancy) and my great Aunt Margeret used to always talk about their favorite horse named "Pepsi".

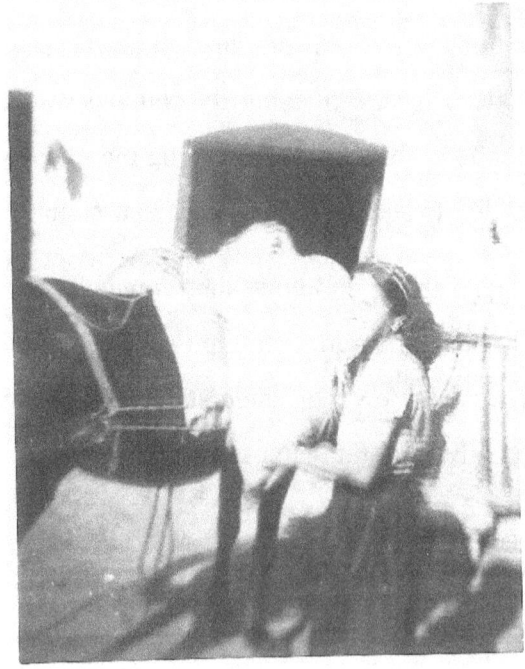

Photo: Great grandmother with Thoroughbred horse

The story of going to the local tennis courts and breaking one of wooden tennis rackets my family had wasn't just a solitary thrust of my strength. It was the new standard in my family's assortment of tennis rackets. Just my mother and father had their own favorite tennis racket and the other tennis rackets were fair game for me to play with. The racket brands we had were Wilson, Dunlop, Spalding, Rawlings, Bancroft, etc. Over the next few years I would end up breaking all of the wooden tennis rackets we had. I remember using wood glue we had around the house and tried to put the pieces back together. The inevitable happened. I was allowed to use my father's Dunlop Max Ply wooden tennis racket. It was a top quality racket for its time and had tight strings. I played with it at the tennis courts with my family. The racket cracked at the base of the frame. After returning home I started to repair the racket very quickly when no one was looking. It was a good patch job and I just left it on a hook in the garage of our house. My father probably knew I cracked the racket but could tell it was from innocent fun, I wasn't to blame. With the wood tennis rackets breaking, I also broke the tennis strings on some of them. I also did a quick fit on these too. Putting the strings back through the holes of the tennis frame, pulling the string and tying a knot at the end.

The string repair worked and the tennis rackets were still playable for a very basic game of tennis. I was learning about tennis rackets all on my own. I was able to see how rackets can get glued together and strings can get pulled and put back into the frame. One day I was inspecting the tennis rackets we owned by the entrance door to the garage, my mother and father walked over and told me that I could play pro tennis if I kept at it. I really started to think about pro tennis as a sport to excel in, it was a great feeling! Trying to figure out who is a pro tennis player and what they're all about, I looked at some of the tennis rackets we owned and noticed names on some of them. I liked looking at two rackets made by Dunlop, one was for a male and the other for a female. They were made as a pair that was sold together. Back then and in the present time, almost all tennis rackets are unisex but this pair was different. I saw the names on the tennis rackets. The female racket was Ms. Evonne Goolagong and the male was Mr. Marty Riessen. I looked at the tennis racket with Mr. Marty Riessen's name on it and noticed his photograph on the frame. I started to wonder about playing pro tennis as great as Mr. Riessen. This started some dreams of making it as a pro tennis player and having a tennis racket made with my name on it.

Our family didn't think about playing tennis every day. When I was young my parents were involved with the Catholic Church and we always went to 12 O'clock Mass on Sunday. They originally met at a church related event with the Knights of Columbus and always stayed involved with this community. Since we moved into a new Subdivision there was an expansion of the population. The Catholic Church had a fundraiser to build a new Parish in the Jericho area. My father always wanted to help and donated money to fill this need. The St. Paul the Apostle Roman Catholic Church was constructed in Brookville, NY adjacent to the Jericho Junior Senior High School. I attended religious education from a young age and became a confirmed Catholic. There was a confirmation ceremony at the same parish and a big party for me at home filled with relatives.

My parents involved our family in things like the Boy Scouts of America. Since I had two older brothers I attended many meetings for 7 years. Many events were held at night and we used to return home at 12:00 am. After I was old enough I joined the Scouts too. This involved attending the group meetings and participating in planned events. Some were competitions where I would get merits and prizes.

We also involved ourselves in an assortment of things like PTA events and Political rallies. These were usually held at the elementary school's meeting room. We also used to attend the Veterans Day parade each year. The parade was right down Broadway passing through the Train Station in Hicksville, NY.

At one Political rally, my father was changing sides in his vote from Republican to Democrat for this election and was backing Mr. Mario Cuomo for Governor of NY. There I met two other boys. They were Andrew and Chris Cuomo. Mr. Mario Cuomo's two sons. We made friends and played kickball in the hallway of the Robert Seaman Elementary School. They could tell in one minute from my athletic sharpness, that I was probably going to play some kind of professional sport.

I was a strong athlete and smart student from the very beginning. In Kindergarten, my test scores made it so I could attend an advanced school in Plainview, NY, and potentially work at the top of the corporate world. I was also told from athletic testing that I could become a professional sports player.

When I graduated kindergarten at the Robert Seaman Elementary School, there was a big ceremony and diplomas were handed out. My father and mother were there to experience this with me. With the whole group of graduating children present, I introduced my father to my new girlfriend Dahlia.

Growing up on Long Island also had a lot of water and beaches close by. There was a nice breeze present and it possessed some challenging weather. We lived in the middle of the island, and experienced the north shore and south shore water lines. My family liked taking a few hours and going to the beach when the weather was good. There were other beach fun activities we frequently did that most people would only participate in on vacation.

Since my father was wounded in WWII he was required to stay at the VA, Veterans Administration, Hospital 2 nights per year. This was a very serious reality I was learning about. The VA always took great care of my father and gave him hope to keep living his life and overcoming his disability. His war wounds were bad enough to have a sticker on his car for disabled veterans. This provided us with a special parking space when we went shopping. Even though he was just an honorably discharged 1st private with a bronze star he was still a part of the organizational structure with the US Army. This was a serious reality about my father's health condition.

The shadow of my father's health complications loomed quietly over our family, yet he never ceased to share his dreams for me. He recognized the talent and intelligence that lay dormant within me even at a young age, often voicing opinions of my potential during my formative years. "One day, you might even play at a pro level," he'd say, a hint of pride lacing his words, even if I was only playing games with neighborhood kids.

But life has a way of changing course with a ferocious force. The excitement of learning to break free with my tennis skills turned into grief and loss when cancer took him from us at too young an age of 8. He was a cigar chain smoker and needed this habit to keep working and living a functional life. It was a devastating blow that reshaped the core of our family dynamics, leaving my mother with a hefty burden and my brothers and I navigating the confusing waters of adolescence without our guiding star.

Yet, in the wake of this devastation, an opportunity arose. Just one year after my father's passing, my mother, determined to honor his dreams for me, searched tirelessly for a new tennis racket — specifically, the Prince racket with this big round head that everyone was talking about in school. When she finally located one at a local sports shop in Hicksville, NY, she brought it home, unaware of the fate that awaited our newest family member. As my small hands gripped the sleek frame, I bent it completely out of shape in enthusiastic swings during the first time I tried out the racket on the tennis court. Cementing my status as a boy who would not be limited by loss or grief.

That bending of the racket, the very embodiment of my journey thus far, would lead me down a path I had not anticipated. My mother's unwavering support led to a big sponsorship opportunity. This happened when my mother Mrs. Rose Riggio returned the racket to the sports shop to ask for a refund or exchange and the owner of S&S Sports shop, Mr. Patrick Mulrooney, looked at the racket and was so amazed at how I had the great strength to bend the frame of the tennis racket. He told my mother that I could make it as a pro tennis player. To back up this observation he decided to sponsor me as a prospective pro tennis player. This included 3 new tennis rackets and a tennis bag. I now officially had a pro contract. The message was passed to me that I need to slowly learn how to play tennis and as I play better and better I will have tournaments to play.

My mother was helping to craft a bridge from the innocence of childhood play to the thrilling world of professional tennis—a world bursting with promise and potential.

The next year in 5th grade there was even more achievement and excitement! I was well-liked in class and was voted the Student Class President. From this, I was greeted by the school's Principal and signed papers for the class.

That year wasn't over yet. My 5th-grade teacher informed us there was a new gym teacher who was brought to the school to teach a special assignment for gymnastics. When he asked who wanted to take these lessons, I quickly raised my hand. All of the students who raised their hands were allowed to take the lessons.

The teacher taught us gymnastics a few times a week for 1 hour. I liked the sport of gymnastics. I started to feel stronger in my body and mind. Meanwhile, the teacher showed me how to use the gymnastics apparatus and I started to improve. Confidence in my skills as a sportsman was growing. The teacher gave everyone a physical gymnastic test. I was growing stronger and I was told my test score is within the range to win a gold medal in the Olympics.

This special school assignment led to a gymnastics demonstration event at night. All of the parents and students were invited. I performed so well in the boys' gymnastics that I was made the winner of the event. The large crowd of parents and teachers were all applauding and cheering for me. As I exited the gymnasium and walked into the hallway, there were so many students and parents cheering me. Some people greeted me with nice words of accomplishment and others asked me to sign my autograph.

A lady from outside the school was there and walked over to me. She informed me that I was just chosen for the Olympic Star Program as a result of my great performance. She told me about how we are going to meet during school classes. From these sessions I will learn how to make a new future for myself.

I went to each meeting and she offered me to travel to California to become great in gymnastics and entertainment. I forwarded this offer to my mother. My mother said no! She didn't believe in the Olympic star program and didn't care about me playing gymnastics.

This experience with the Olympic star program wasn't a waste of time. Everyone around me knew I was picked for greatness and I always met other Gymnast's since that time.

As I reflect upon these formative years, I see a narrative unfolding, woven with laughter, teachings, and family history, as well as the burgeoning realization of a dream that would become my lifeblood. It is within this narrative that the essence of my identity was born. With each serve and smash on the court, I ultimately took steps not just toward athletic triumph but also toward honoring my father's legacy of honesty and integrity. And so, this is where my story begins — at the intersection of passion, family, and an unyielding desire to carve my path in the world of tennis.

Chapter Two
The Rise of a Tennis Dream

There was something so surreal about the idea of being a sponsored player; I was just an ordinary kid, yet here was the potential for a future in professional tennis. With Mr. Mulrooney's support, it was possible to make it big in pro tennis.

Thus began my journey. From the directive from Mr. Patrick Mulrooney, I had to figure out how to improve my tennis playing and get noticed to play tennis tournaments. In my first year in middle school, the teachers explained there was an assortment of clubs available. I asked around for a tennis club but there were none available. So I talked to some of my school mates and they wanted to play tennis too.

I devised an idea of how to put players together to have a match of tennis. My ideas really worked and the pool of players started to grow. We were playing during school and after school. The only problem was the Jericho Junior Senior High School had a policy of students playing unattended. This means the school had to have one teacher oversee the activity. The school contacted me through my friends and they told me the school's athletic administrator Mr. Anthony Cambria has to run our tennis club. I agreed and I was made club president and my friend Karenga Smith was made the vice president.

Our new coach Mr. Anthony Cambria started to organize the tennis matches. I was really amazed that the games were very similar to what I had arranged. They were well-matched games. Mr. Cambria came out to the tennis courts and played some tennis with me. He tested my abilities by asking me to hit the ball in certain locations on the court. He was very impressed and wanted me to strive even further. In the following weeks, he recommended I go to the library and read books about how to play tennis. He gave me some book titles to search for. I was trying hard to play better.

My winning percentage started at 50 percent, I used to calculate the matches I won versus the matches I lost. As I played the club tennis matches directed by Mr. Camria, I played one older student. He was an excellent tennis player and I was trying to keep up my playing against him. After the match we talked and he knew I was the president of the club. He suggested that I need to play the best of all the members in his opinion. I started to think about what he said and worked on improving my tennis playing even more. I read more books on playing tennis in the local public library and started to hit some balls on my own to improve my tennis serve and other precision shots. My playing did start to improve. I started to win more matches and after this new push at improving my tennis game my percentage of winning improved to 75 percent. I played the older student again and won the match. He was shocked and yet happy. I told him I took his suggestion seriously and started to play better. After my percentage increased to 75 percent there was no turning back to playing great tennis.

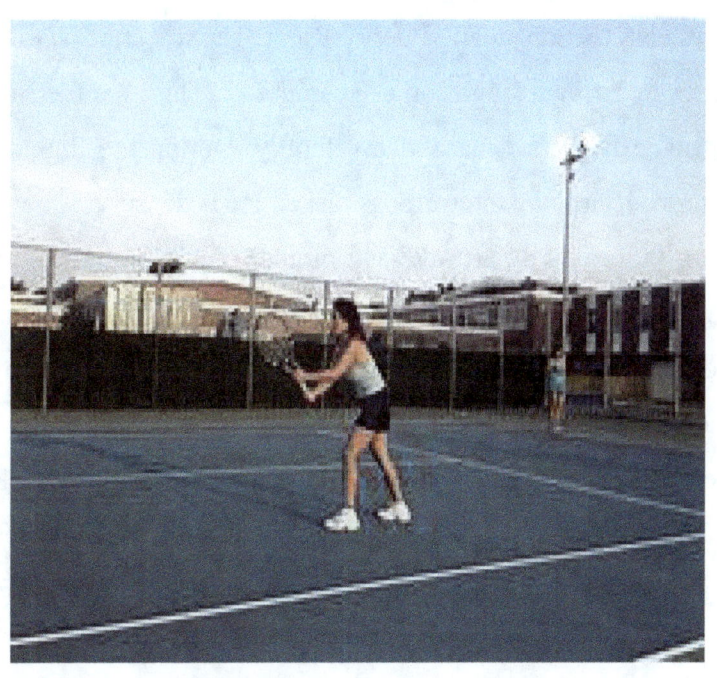

Photo: Jericho Junior Senior School Tennis Courts

As my playing improved Mr. Cambria had me play some kids that weren't going to the school. A short time later, he asked me to meet him at his office. He declared I was playing excellent tennis and he thought I could make it as a pro tennis player. Showing me some papers, Anthony made an offer for me to sign a pro contract with the National Tennis Center. I agreed and signed the papers.

Along with the signing, Mr. Cambria explained I would receive a vacation. In just a few days my mother received the phone call and she agreed to take a 3-day vacation to San Juan, Puerto Rico. The vacation started with an airplane flight on a Boeing 747. This was the first airplane flight for me and my family. During the flight to Puerto Rico, the stewardess asked "whose servicemen's family are you a part of?" My mother didn't know what to say. The stewardess explained the flight is only for government family members and USA servicemen. As my mother wondered about her reservations, I decided to tell her. I explained that I signed a contract to play pro tennis with Mr. Anthony Cambria and the National Tennis Center. I am now a member of the USA government. My mother Rose was so amazed she informed the stewardess right away about my tennis playing. As we exited the airplane after landing in San Juan, Puerto Rico. The stewardess crew asked about each member of our family. She called on the telephone and verified I was the USA member that made the trip possible. We were on a very nice vacation and returned without any problems.

After returning home from the vacation, I continued to play more tennis matches. I stopped in Mr. Cambria's office and he was ecstatic about my tennis playing. I played a series of tennis matches and made it past the ITF level tennis, and the minor leagues, and made it to the junior ATP. This is the major league of tennis. It wasn't easy to win these matches. I really had to focus my mind to achieve even higher than before. The extra effort to win these matches became the standard in my playing.

From this great tennis success, it was time to select a player's name. He explained the name was like an actor's stage name. I could use the name in public and I don't have to reveal my natural name. This would provide me with safety and security. It was also to remove people's prejudice from my heritage. I was asked to think of a player name for myself. I returned back with some proposed names. Some of the names were John Arrow, John Stare, John Tops, John Ridge, John McCullen, John Liner, etc. Mr. Cambria was required to call the ATP on the phone and have my new name approved. After a few rejections, I finally requested the name Jack Racet. This name was approved.

Just a few weeks later I rode my bicycle to the local Mall. I liked to go to the Broadway Mall in Hicksville, NY. It was just a 15-minute bike ride away. This time the trip to the Mall was different. I was starting to use my new name Jack Racet. At the entrance to the Mall, there was a girl my own age. She asked me if I could help her repair her broken bicycle. I obliged and was able to fix her bicycle in a few minutes. She was really happy about it and we talked for a few minutes. She told me that her name was Dahlia and I told her my name was Jack. We exchanged phone numbers and started to make friends.

We did all of the usual things together like riding bicycles and going to the game room in the Mall. Me and Dahlia took to dating quickly and when I told her about my pro tennis playing she was very excited. She told me about her ice skating with Dorothy Hamill's Ice Capades. We were both in the entertainment world at that point.

From visiting Dahlia at her home I was able to meet her mother and father. Dahlia's father told me he was born in Shanghai, China and used to play ITF tennis and liked the idea of me and Dahlia getting married together. Her mother came from an Italian heritage and was very nice introducing herself. At this time, Dahlia told me she was recently voted the Beauty Queen at a local pageant. Me and Dahlia scheduled one day of the week in the evening hours to regularly meet at her house. This kind of meeting would go on for a long time. The one thing about Dahlia was her parents weren't thinking about her feelings and used her. Dahlia ran up a bill buying clothing at one of the shops in the Mall. Her parents didn't want to pay the bill. Instead, I went to the store with Dahlia and they told me she owed $200 in clothing. They planned to cause Dahlia big problems with the law over her open balance. I took some of my savings from home and paid her bill. The situation calmed down. At her house, she had plans for us to get married and she hoped my pro tennis would keep us together. I agreed and we were unofficially engaged.

Dahlia was the same young girl from Kindergarten. The school district had different school locations and after Kindergarten she attended another public school. She also was the only female in the school district to make the Olympic star program in gymnastics. Since we attended different middle and high schools we would meet at her house or the Broadway Mall. We liked the game room and made other friends there to play with. Dahlia introduced me to her friend Annette. She was another ice skater and liked to play video games. We made friends and the three of us played together. After the game room went out of business, Dahlia took a job at Auntie Anne's kiosk in the Mall. You could buy soft pretzels and a soft drink there. This new job helped stop a problem with her parents. Dahlia's mother was monitoring the telephone at home and it was difficult to contact her. Dahlia's new job helped to circumvent this problem.

Filled with the sweet symphony of tennis balls hitting against rackets, the thrill of competition, and the camaraderie of friends who shared in my passion. As I transitioned from my tennis club to playing pro tennis matches. So, in a moment of brilliance and with a few enthusiastic friends, we gathered to take a leap into the world of competition and play.

A new friend I made playing tennis was Ms. Heidi Stanton. She was on the school tennis team and was also playing under the direction of Mr. Anthony Cambria. From this common coach, the three of us used to talk together in public school.

My singles playing improved to where I was already the number one player this included the varsity tennis team. I was the de facto tennis team captain. I turned the position down and just played pro singles. This was the correct decision and Heidi started to help me with my pro tennis instead of just school tennis. We played tennis together. She was very smart and a certified tennis trainer. She could gauge my playing level. She saw me pass the team test and the 5.5 test to play national tournament-level tennis.

Aside from tennis Heidi used to ice skate at the local indoor ring. She told me stories of vying for the Olympic trials in ice skating. Julie Stein was Heidi's friend and she was also a member of the school tennis team. The three of us used to hit the ball together as a warm-up. In addition, Julie was another ice skater and to my surprise both Heidi and Julie knew my girlfriend Dahlia from ice skating with Dorothy Hamill. One amazing fact is all of my female skating friends performed as the Smurfs in the Dorothy Hamill's Ice Capades show.

My ability to play great tennis was powered by my great physical health. I was always exercising in some way. Living in the suburbs allowed me to ride my bicycle to friends' houses or to the local tennis courts. There were open school yards and public parks where I could assemble friends to play different popular sports like American football, baseball/softball, basketball, etc. My neighborhood friends would invite me to join in the same sports. These kinds of physical activities would happen after-school on the weekends and after night fall under the lights too. I was staying in great shape.

At this age, I used to read a lot of books. Even years earlier I was the number one reader in the book club at the Jericho Public Library. I liked to read autobiographies and learn how individuals grew up and advanced in life. I liked to read the periodicals in the school library before classes started in my public school. The library was open early when the buses arrived at the junior-senior high school.

In sixth grade, during a career day at Robert Seaman Elementary School, I found myself faced with a pivotal decision. The guest speaker guided my classmates and me through various career possibilities, encouraging us to reflect on our own strengths and ambitions. Initially, I proposed becoming a Lawyer to the speaker; however, as the presentation unfolded and aligned with my aptitude, the advice shifted toward becoming an Architect. The notion of working with design and building construction captivated my imagination, igniting a passion that would shape the course of my life.

By the time I entered middle school, I immersed myself in a robust educational environment that nurtured my burgeoning interest in architecture. My school district provided valuable resources, including drafting classes and various art courses. I diligently explored every opportunity laid before me, knowing that each class helped lay the groundwork for my future.

As I transitioned from elementary school to middle school, personal computers began to permeate education.

Intrigued by technology, I considered this emerging career path, maybe even embarking on a journey as a software developer, etc. I took all of the computer classes my school had available. I even had a summer job with the computer department assembling the new order of Apple PC's.

To continue my career search, there was a special class available to learn how to fly an airplane. The class was called Aviation Operations. There was a 7-year waiting list for this class. Me and a couple of my friends used to check-in to keep our names on the waiting list. I was finally able to attend the class in my senior year of high school. The class was part of a technical school district run by the New York State Department of Education. I took a school bus from my high school to the class located on the Grumman defense property in Bethpage, NY. There I was able to excel at the ground school. I was also involved in student government as a class representative. The class comprised the top students from the County. Many of the kids were graduating as the Valedictorians of their High School. There were piloting instructors at an offsite business located at the Republic Airport, Farmingdale, NY. The company was commissioned by the School District. I learned to pilot single-engine land aircraft. They were the high-wing Cessna 152 and Cessna 172, and the low-wing

Grumman American Cheetah and Grumman American Tiger, the Tiger was a slightly larger airplane. One flight instructor said I was his best pilot of his whole career. This was from a Veteran WWII pilot. I earned straight A's in the class and graduated with the Outstanding Student Award. On the first try, I passed my flight test in the spring of 1997. I was then given my license certificate to pilot on my own.

What also came out of the exciting education was my flight doctor. To fly an airplane I needed a physical exam. My doctor Robert DiPasca who was approved by the FAA also had a history of medical excellence. He was trained by the U.S. armed forces and examined many servicemen. Dr. DiPasca also worked as a sports doctor. He was the doctor for some known sports players.

Dr. DiPasca gave me a thorough physical exam. This included a blood test. After I returned to his office, he told me I was In excellent physical condition. Not only that, I had the best physical shape he ever met in his whole career in my weight class. He was very impressed. He took my test report and put it on the wall.

On August 1, 1986, I was 149 lbs, Pressure 114/74, Pulse 70, Hearing 15/15, Vision 20/20. And 3% body fat and had very low cholesterol. I was 5'11".

The previous report he removed from the wall was a US Marine. Dr. DiPasca Already had many years of experience and was planning his retirement in a few years. During my tennis-playing years, I had to visit his office a few times for sports injuries. I had some very painful injuries and thought they were really bad. I was concerned they were going to become permanent. He told me what the name of each injury was and explained how to prevent further sports injuries. I was lucky when Dr. DiPasca explained tennis injuries can heal on their own. I can just let my body heal slowly and I will return to full health.

Tennis was my best sport and just by chance, I played on the school track team. I wasn't the best at the track. I played the 100-yard dash. One thing the participants started to notice about me was I always lead the race at the 10 yard mark. From this astonishing fact the team had students and coaches watch this during each race. This was another reason tennis was my best sport. The tennis court measures just about 10 yards from the baseline to the net.

All these tennis endeavors led to my advancement in pro tennis. My new pro tennis life off the court was starting to grow. I was making new friends and people really liked the name Jack. It was an adventurous name and proved to give me a new and uncharted course for myself. This new adventure was backed by Anthony Cambria's unwavering encouragement. He believed in me, and with newfound support, I was stepping onto the path of possible greatness. The only greatness I had to leave behind was my player name Jack Racet. Mr. Cambria told me the name wasn't registering well in public. The core reason was when I made my new place in the local Mall, no-one really knew who Jack Racet was or where he lived. Instead of working out these details and legalizing the name or just keeping the name on the tennis courts, like some people suggested, the player name Jack Racet was ended! Mr. Cambria apologized to me that the player name wasn't working out well, he acknowledged these unforeseen problems were already erupting for my pro life. In an effort to correct the name problem, he called the ATP office and tried some new names. The name the person suggested was John Holton. This instantly became my new player name and was recorded with the ATP.

The new name was a flop. Most people didn't like it. Some coaches wouldn't write the name John Holton down. This was frustrating and most people just knew my first name John. To see if there was a loophole in player names I tried a few others while introducing myself to a tennis opponent. One was the name Amadeus. This name was good. Some kids liked it, they thought it was funny and playful. Maybe an important name? This name eventually faded away and was replaced with new player names.

My overall tennis ability and form started to advance. I started to have a strict routine of entering the tennis courts, doing ten push-ups and a series of stretches for the muscles in my body before the matches started. My serve advanced to where my opponent would have to think twice before deciding to serve first. This started to happen when my opponent would serve a ball to me and I would hit it right down the line and would pass the baseline before he could make a grab at the ball. If my opponent was on the right side of his court I would hit the ball to the left side and vice versa. After breaking the spirit of my opponent by having an amazing return of his serve. I would usually start with a series of ace serves to start the first game. I didn't ram the ball down the court the whole match. The next set of hits I would work on were some cross court shots deep, cross court shots short, lob shots, and net shots. My playing was so amazing I ended up giving one game away to my opponent. I usually did this first and foremost in my tennis club. This is because the participants would start to complain that I was winning all of the games. I started to feel the telephone ringing at home after these blow out games. The same rule started to apply to my pro matches. Some players would become vocal and say that even in the pros a game could become mismatched. They would opt out to play in a lower tournament instead of me winning so big.

The word of my tennis playing successes was reaching my sponsor Mr Patrick Mulrooney of S&S Sports. I talked to Mr. Mulrooney and he told me it was time for me to have a tennis racket brand sponsor. To have this kind of sponsor each prospective company would send a scout to watch my tennis matches at the courts in Jericho.

As I played the matches during the upcoming weeks, I would see someone sitting near the courts. I talked to Mr. Mulrooney after the review process was over. He told me about each company; Babolat, Wilson, Gamma, Prince, etc. The Prince Racket Company selected me for sponsorship. A few days later I was given 2 Prince rackets to go along with my pro stock tennis racket. I was given a new bag, sweats, Prince Sneakers, etc. The Prince Racket representative came to the court side and congratulated me. He gave me some Prince-printed items including individual tennis racket head covers and stickers that are affixed to the racket frame. I was to use these advertising tools and he asked me to display them during the matches. He explained I should always have the Prince name shown for advertising purposes.

The coordination between my coach Anthony Cambria, my sports shop sponsor Patrick Mulrooney, and my racket brand Prince racket started to work perfectly. There were no disputes and each party wanted to invest more, more, and even more. With each tournament I played—the Manhattan Open, the American Airlines tournament, the Eastern tournament —I garnered recognition. I was no longer that bewildered child holding a bent aluminum racket; I was forging my path into adulthood as a tennis player. I balanced academics, friendships, and my newfound responsibilities as a star tennis player. By now, I had honed my craft to earn respect among my peers and newer players alike.

Thus, my story ramped toward its circle, with Patrick, Anthony and Prince championing me as I began to bridge the rift between childhood and professional athlete. There was a relentless awe in my heart now as I pursued dreams that felt both tangible and nebulous. I found community in the courts, hope in the skies, and the promise of competition in my feet. My journey to stardom was just beginning, fueled by the will to succeed—woven from the magic of childhood hope and glowing with ambition.

Chapter Three
The Courts of Triumph

As the sun hung high in the sky, casting a golden hue over the Jericho Junior Senior High School tennis courts, I felt an exhilarating sense of ownership wash over me. I could still hear the echoes of the countless matches I played there, each point won and lost forging my resolve. It was on these courts where I first asserted myself, and where my journey from a novice player to a contender truly began. With every swing of my racket, I saw my previously modest winning percentage lift itself, from a shaky 50% to an impressive 75% with an ultimate 96%. Each match strengthened not only my skills but also my identity as a player.

In time, those very courts became my sanctum. They were no longer merely places to practice; they were mine—my stage, if you will. As my victories mounted, my coach named me "the Johnny Show". As the students and teachers loved to see me play tennis from the school room windows. Defending my position grew into a badge of honor, as the other players soon learned that stepping onto my court meant facing a formidable opponent. Slowly but surely, my connection to tennis solidified, and with each match I played, my confidence surged.

Mr. Anthony Cambria, my coach and steadfast source of encouragement, was always by my side, watching my ascent with a mixture of pride and anticipation. He saw in me what I was beginning to grasp: the potential for a professional tennis career. It was this foresight that led us to formalize our partnership—contract signed, commitment forged. Not too long afterward, my sponsorship with Patrick Mulrooney and S&S Sports flourished, leading to a lucky break. Patrick introduced me to a stream of seasoned players—all coming through the National Tennis Center or going to matches in various venues across New York.

With this influx of competitors, I quickly found myself in a whirlwind of exhilarating matches, learning from and facing pros who had already made a name for themselves. It was thrilling and nerve-wracking all at the same time. However, the surge in competition only fueled my ambition, and my winning percentage climbed higher and higher. The courts at Jericho had become a revered hallowed ground for me—a place where triumphs melded with dreams.

My tennis club was still playing the whole time as I played pro tennis. My club tennis matches hid my pro tennis matches because students and teachers would see 2 tennis players on the court. They couldn't tell the level of the match. The tennis players in the club improved with me as a player. No match was easy to win. I always had to play my best match to win. The tennis club had a year-end tournament In 11th grade. I won the tournament. In 12th grade, my playing spectators grew and I won the final match. With three stories of school rooms filled with students and teachers watching. It was even videotaped by the school staff. I won the final point on a hot sun-filled afternoon. As I exited the tennis court I walked to the school hallway doors. There I met a crowd of cheering students and teachers. They all grabbed me and asked me to sign tennis balls. I obliged with my signatures. It was a very memorable afternoon.

Back at my coach's office with Mr. Anthony Cambria, the talk shifted to pro tennis. He started to update me with my tournament wins. He told me I won the junior ATP tournament called ABN. For this victory there was a nice size trophy. A took some pictures of me holding the trophy. This was becoming a new standard for me. When Mr. Cambria received the trophies for my tournament wins I would meet him at his office and have a trophy photo taken. In some trophy photos, my friend Heidi was there to witness this exciting event. She was very happy and was always rooting for me to win more pro matches. My junior pro tournament wins were growing. This is for kids under the age of 18. On some tournament wins, like the Eastern Tournament, he would get honored by how he was the coach for a big winning player. I already knew from the opponents I played that I was listed as the number 1 ranked player as a junior. Mr. Cambria told me the same. He also added that I won the Most Valuable Player as a junior player in the ATP. He also took records of my other playing statistics. I have many ATP records for my tennis playing.

Mr. Cambria was a pro tennis player when he was younger. He taught me that a pro tennis player's career can just stop. He told me to always be prepared for this horror. Mr. Cambria also attended college for athletics education. He earned a master's degree in this field and was studying for a PHD. He worked at my public school as the athletic administrator and was also employed as a tennis

Administrator at the National Tennis Center. He was winning big with coaching my pro tennis career.

Looking to the future, Mr. Cambria, applied for me to attend Clemson University in South Carolina. This was a College that had a pro track for tennis players. The College was also interested in me just playing tennis. I didn't have to attend academic classes. I was accepted into the College in 1984. I talked to the admissions department on the telephone and they were happy to talk to me. They told me my natural name was perfect for pro tennis and they were backing this name. Clemson even suggested using a made up name for my personal life and finances. They knew everyone was going to have a side job and home life. There were some serious legal complexities with the alias names. They also set up an appointment for me to attend the orientation event at the college. As time approached to attend this event, my mother turned down this future. She told me it was too far away for me. She suggested I don't go to college for the first year. My mother never attended college when she was young. I would later get Clemson University's support for my tennis playing.

As I turned 18 years old I also grew into an adult player. My junior years are over and my pro tennis ranking has to now switch to an adult player. My coach, Mr. Cambria, checked my ranking conversion, and I was ranked the 500th player in the adult ATP. I was still able to hold my own court at Jericho High School. This special situation to hold your own court in the adult ATP does happen on occasion. To start off my coach told me I was to play on my court at a certain time after school.

The date had arrived. I waited on my court and an adult player from the National Tennis Center arrived in his car. As he arrived, so did the CBS Sports news van. CBS is a franchise of broadcast television stations that have national and local news. In NYC they were Channel 2. It had a camera boom on top of the van. I started to play the new opponent in a warm-up match. I looked and saw the camera boom go up in the air. My opponent didn't want to lose. As he ran to the net I hit the ball over his head. He ran to his left then I hit the ball past his right. He ended up falling down on the floor. He was only 32 years old. I was to find out his name was Vitas, the captain of the pro players at the National Tennis Center. The news van drove away. From that meeting, I was asked to show up at the same court after school at certain times of the week.

I started to play warm-up matches and ATP tour matches. All of the top pro players in the ATP started to play a match with me on my court. I started to win big. My Coach Mr. Cambria told me the tennis Head Coach at the National Tennis Center, Harry, has assigned me a tennis instructor. The new tennis instructor was directed to have me learn the required nomenclature of adult pro tennis playing.

I met with the instructor on the tennis courts and started to learn all of the new requirements. Some things I learned didn't fit my 80s-style tennis playing. Overall I excelled at learning the requirements and was really achieving. I started to apply these new tools in the ATP tour matches he oversaw. I was starting to advance in the adult pros. As I played pros people watched on TV, I started to experience my opponents wanting to make deals. This was another lesson I had to get through. The answer was no deals, just win each game.

The fact that I was the world star player was evident. All of the players were coming to play me and the chances of them winning were very small. I had just turned 18 years old and even though I was winning there were many levels and ranking numbers to move up to. My ranking jumped to

250. Some players were already at rank 1. One player from Australia was Mr. Brad Drewett. He was one of few tennis players like myself who had his own court in previous years. As I won matches the other veteran players started to get the idea that I wasn't going to fall apart and lose. They started to compare me with American-born Mr. Brian Gottfried. He was another player who held his own court and played the best tournaments.

As the male pros came to my tennis court, so did the female players. They used to bus the players from the National Tennis Center in Flushing, NYC to my court. I usually just warmed up with the females. I played a few matches against the female players. I was able to win all of the matches against the female players. I never lost a pro tennis match against a female player in my whole career.

The other players were used to coming to my Tennis Court at the Jericho Junior Senior High School. Since I was sponsored by Prince Tennis rackets they felt comfortable using the name "Beast" before someone played a match against me. The Prince Racket Company has a popular tennis racket called "the Beast". The term "the Beast man" was also used. The new nickname grew. This idea of a beast on the court made people wonder if I was starting to dominate my tennis game.

There was suddenly a horrible tragedy at the National Tennis Center. The Head Coach Harry suddenly died of Cancer. He already knew about my career as a junior player and had communicated with Mr. Anthony Cambria about my transition from junior pro tennis to adult pro tennis. Harry approved of everyone coming to play at my court. I saw the Head Coaches last day visiting the Jericho courts. He waved goodbye to everyone and drove away. The other players involved were afraid this was like my father dying to me. There was a period of instability to see who the next Head Coach was and if I was going to stay in good favor. Everything worked out great with the next Head Coach, Bid, introducing himself to me at my court.

The next parameter of pro tennis was the tennis agility test. This is a standardized test that is given to all new pro players. I took the test and scored the best score to date. This surpassed the other top scores of some active players. This started to make these other players jealous. My top score made the other players believe I am a top player and that is why they are coming to my court. They must have been unaware that I was already the number 1 junior player and won many top ATP tennis tournaments.

The pro-playing continued through the winter. I made the rank of the 100th player. My tennis instructor was switched to another top player. They both called on the phone and submitted requests for my name and tennis rank to get published. They were already giving me ideas of having a publicist and agent.

One thing I discovered playing tennis at my adult age of 18 years old was there were many pro tennis players piloting single engine land airplanes. Many players took to this adventure of flight in small aircraft. Many players already had their pilot's license to take the yoke of control and commandeer their own path in the air. They even used to fly out of the same airport Farmingdale, NY on Long Island. As I was allowed to fly solo at that time, I used to see many pro players in their Cessna, Piper or Grumman American airplanes on the taxiways waiting for takeoff. There were two large runways at the airport for a mix of recreational and commercial plane traffic. The other sports players used to wave over when they recognized me, I used to wave back in reply. It was an exhilarating feeling to share the same interests of aviation and sports. It was an amazing coincidence that sports players found their way to pilot small airplanes. I was wondering if the ability to play sports were connected to the skills you need to pilot an airplane. This could involve having great reflexes with coordination and the concentration to pilot the airplane, you also have to pass the flight medical exam. Possessing the great desire to achieve could also contribute to this kind of ability. To conduct recreational flying there was some money you had to pay to use the airplanes, along with training and legal papers. It wasn't a low cost hobby. With flying you needed to drive your car to the airport. This is part of the lingo in the suburbs. Having a nice stylish car to drive helps too. Overall, this kind of venture does keep you with a progressive group of people. Piloting isn't very social in the air but it was very challenging. I originally pursued this adventure as a career idea. The job to just locate passengers' luggage at the airport was good enough for me. I was starting to think people who pilot airplanes somehow could keep their pro tennis careers alive, but it wasn't true. You don't need to take high risks on the side to play pro tennis. I found this out a few years later.

Playing the other adult pros was very intense. The ball hitting was very fast and required great strength and ability. The one thing that started to happen was my tennis racket was breaking as I hit the ball. I would break as many as 3 rackets in one match. I had my mother bring the broken rackets back to my pro shop. Mr. Mulrooney replaced each racket quickly. He said each racket was covered with his insurance. The word coming back from the Prince Racket Company was they were very impressed with the broken rackets. I even talked to the Prince Company representative and he asked me about the tennis racket frame.

My playing continued and I started to play adult tournaments. I started to win tournaments. At this time I was selected to play the National Tournament. I was still holding my own court and they allowed the matches to play out on my court. These matches were on the weekend, usually Saturday morning and sometimes on Sunday. I started to play the tournament matches and won big. The organizer was really impressed with my playing. I was playing so amazing he asked me to play 2 matches each Saturday. I was usually returning home with 2 wins.

During the National Tournament, my matches were seen on television via a sports news van with a camera boom. The television broadcast was confirmed by my neighbor as I returned home. Mr. Hy Ozer, a school principal, always walked out of his house and congratulated me - telling me he saw me win the tennis match on television. I won 4 parts of the National Tournament with trophies in my season segment. I also had the highest number of points in the USA. From this I was the number 1 player entering the next tournament, the Davis Cup. Prince Tennis Racket Company was ecstatic at this time and started to buy more into my contract.

The National Tournament organizer, Bob, was also the sole manager for selecting the US Olympic Team. I was invited to play in the next Olympics. Tennis was returning to the Olympics and he was filling the list with the top pros like myself. I said OK to join the US Olympic team. The only problem was he asked if I made more than $3,000 in equipment, clothes, or cash and I said yes. Just my Adidas sweat suit was $3,000 from Patrick Mulrooney's sports shop. This honesty paid off because the other pros played in the Olympics and were caught later as illegal players. They were convicted in a US Court and sentenced to the San Quentin Prison for 6 months because they lied to the Olympics that they were Amateur players.

The National Tournament playing didn't get past my girlfriend Dahlia. I was updating her on my playing as we met at her parents' house late in the evening. She was so excited about it. I told her when I was playing a tennis match and she showed up to watch. One time she brought Ms. Dorothy Hamill, her friend from Ice Capades, and they watched me win another match. At this time I was able to play a tennis match against Mr. Dean Paul Martin, actor Dean Martin's son. I won the match and coincidentally I won all of the matches Dahlia watched.

In my earliest memories of stepping onto a tennis court, my father's words echoed in my mind: "Always play fair, never cheat." This principle became the bedrock of my character as I developed my skills, honed my techniques, and prepared to compete at the highest levels of tennis. However, as I transitioned into professional matches, the stark reality surfaced: not everyone shared this commitment to integrity. The world of tennis I had entered was a complex landscape, marred by dishonesty and unethical practices that threatened the very spirit of the game.

As I encountered my fellow competitors, I began to observe behaviors that betrayed my father's teachings. Cheating was not an isolated issue but rather a systematic challenge that some players engaged in with alarming frequency. This was not merely about misjudging a ball's landing; it involved a whole host of tactics designed to manipulate outcomes in their favor. From calling balls out that were clearly in, to switching scores of games mid-match, 4-2 would get switched to 2-4. I witnessed athletes bending the rules to the point of breaking them entirely.

Moreover, the insidious cry of "out" could also become a weapon in the hands of crafty competitors. In matches where the margin was very thin, these players cleverly exploited the uncertainty surrounding calls. Even with certified umpires present, they could sway judgment through intimidation or sheer audacity. Too often, I noticed that officials, under pressure, would hesitate to overrule a player's claims, allowing the cheaters to prevail. This reliance on the subjective judgment of officials blurred the lines of accountability; I wondered how anyone could reasonably challenge the integrity of the tournament when those enforcing the rules were readily fooled.

From my interactions with players, I learned that cheating was not confined to the present. Many individuals who engaged in such practices had cultivated a history of wrongdoing, often passing down methods to younger players in a misguided attempt to teach them survival in a ruthless sport. This was instead of sharing tips on improving skills through hard practice. Some players would admit to getting taught how to cheat, and acclaim their success in conducting this behavior. The coaches instructing players on how to deceive the system continued their process because it was difficult for most players to contest a match. The players most likely to excel at cheating were players vying to work as group coaches.

Drugs, too, posed a critical threat to the integrity of tennis. Players might resort to performance-enhancing drugs to gain an edge, believing they could sprint faster, hit harder, and endure grueling matches with reckless energy. I could see my competitors using substances that would amplify their performance just enough to push them past tiredness or fatigue. They were caught many times and our match had to get canceled, they would also register my opponent's match as a loss.

Despite the pervasive atmosphere of cheating, the tide began to shift as accountability became crucial. The investigation into fraudulent scoring and the testing for drug usage, but the catch-and-release nature of these offenses created a frustrating dilemma.

Since I was graduating from the Jericho Junior Senior High School in the spring of 1986 I would have to say goodbye to my own court at the school and make my way to a new playing adventure. My player ranking was upgraded to 26 at this time. I was invited to play at the National Tennis Center in Flushing, NYC. They just needed me to show up on my own and start playing.

I encountered some difficulty getting on the courts in Flushing. The doors were locked and the invitation to start playing was still pending. After some months of trying to figure out how to enter the door of the National Tennis Center, I finally did. I called some superiors in the government and the door wax opened for me. So one day I put my tennis bag in the truck of my car and drove to the National Tennis Center. My new parking space was only for top players. I got out of my car and was greeted by the Captain of the pro tennis players named Vitas.

It was an electrifying day when I found myself stepping into the iconic facility, my heart racing with possibility. There, I was given the use of Court 33, a space distinct and vital—a hub for aspiring champions in the Borough of Queens. The court looked worn out with cracks and dim lines defining the playing area. This was the same for the 5 other adjacent courts to fill. My presence made a big difference with improvement of the allotted tennis courts. The courts were quickly renovated with a new hard surface added, along with new nets and posts. There were also brand new gleaming bleachers installed surrounding the tennis courts. To boot, the court's ownership was officially joined with the National Tennis Center's boundaries as I started playing. They were no longer practice courts that were borrowed from the city park. Every time I stepped onto Court 33, it felt like stepping onto a stage with the world as my audience, full of expectation.

After 2 weeks of training and warmup matches, I started to play the ATP pro tour. I started to win big at my own court 33. My great playing had quickly returned from graduation. This was a new advancement for me to keep my same winning ways at a new location. There was no turning back from the previous court I held for many years.

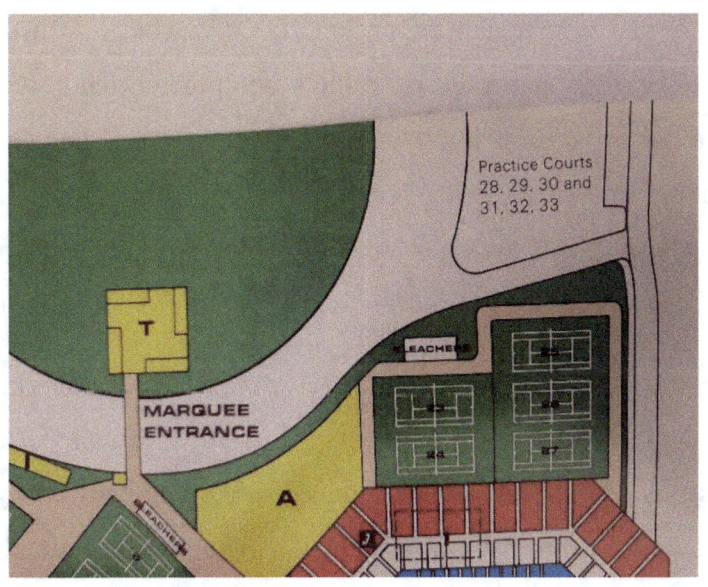

Photo: Map of National Tennis Center showing Court #33.

The other pro players didn't have their own court. Some players waited in their cars located on the opposite side of the tennis center. Some shared the courts in the Green colored out building and some were learning in a group inside a tennis bubble.

As my match-winning continued, my ranking jumped to 17 then 9 then 4. At the National Tennis Center, teams of players from each country would stop in to get their ATP tennis ranking. The Australian team was one of them. The players from Australia also walked to my court 33 to play a match. Two older players Tony Roche and Ken Rosewall both played a match on my court. Of course, I won the matches but they both gave me some pointers on how to play tennis. Tony Roche filled in anything he thought I should improve. He also taught me about the tennis world. His last advice was for me to develop my own playing strategy. With this added knowledge I was to move up to the top ranking.

My court 33 was the dream Mr. Anthony Cambria, Mr. Patrick Mulrooney, and the Prince Racket Company always hoped for. Now familiar with playing at a new location, the future of my pro tennis career was very bright. I could sense that whatever was coming next—each match, each tournament, the new court —would propel me toward the horizon. It wasn't just about being the star player, it was about embracing the journey of all those who sought to rise alongside me. I was ready to confront the future—the courts awaited, alive with promise and possibilities yet untold.

Chapter Four
My Own Tennis Center

From the great success of attaining my own tennis court #33, was my fast move up the rankings. The written ranking of #4 at the National Tennis Center started to build up an urgency to keep moving up. The National Tennis Center head coach of the players, Bid, was in front of my court. He told me he was waiting for me to become such a great tennis player that I could come out and play the tournaments like a "raging bull". He approved my court #33 and knew I would grow to win big in the tournaments.

Bid was the head coach at the National Tennis Center and under him was the Captain of the players, Vitas. I already knew Vitas since I turned 18 years old and started playing with the adult pros. He always told me what the gossip was going around the courts. Vitas started to allude that as my tennis ranking moved up so did the resistance to my playing. There were pressures in the sports business and jealousy rising again.

I finally reached a calm period of time at court #33. The Captain, Vitas, decided to allow some top American College and ITF players to come to the tennis center. Their supporters had submitted requests to have their young players get a try out to play the ATP. Their supporters all had to pay a large fee to play in this try-out. I was the top pro tennis player they were going to meet. As the weeks went by, I played the number 1 collegiate player in the USA and the number 1 ITF player. There were also other top players who wanted a tryout. At the end of this tryout period I was to select one of the players to advance to play the ATP tour.

I won all of the matches against the contestants the Captain sent me. I was an outstanding player to them and they told me they were all grateful to play me. After finishing this run of matches, Vitas asked me who my choice was and I selected the player that was playing the best game. He turned out to be of good character too, as I was told of his progress. This player was a good choice and he remained an ATP player for a number of years. The Captain also chose one player to continue to the ATP tour.

My great playing ability, my judgment of my opponents' playing, and my know-how to win matches and tournaments weren't enough. The Captain of the pros at the National Tennis Center, Vitas, told me I needed more authority to play at the National Tennis Center in Flushing, NY. He asked me if I knew any relatives in high places like nobility. I told him about my grandparents' heritage and he said ok. He would ask inside the main office. Unknown at that time, but important to know now, was the Association of Tennis Professionals, the ATP was owned by people living in the United Arab Emirates, UAE.

Vitas told me that my heritage story checked out and someone was coming to my court. The new visit was from the Prince of Savoy, Mr. Filiberto Emanuele, currently the Prince of Venice. He arrived with his wife Princess Vittoria and his Parents Mr. Vittorio Emanuele, Prince of Naples and Princess Marina. They just flew in from Europe especially for this meeting.

They brought with them the pro tennis player Mr. Sergio Tacchini. He is a well-known player and even has a line of tennis rackets and sports clothes named after him. As the royals watched from the bleachers, I played a tennis match against Mr. Tacchini on court #33. They applauded my tennis playing and were cheering at some of my shots.

The Prince and his family were very impressed to see me win the match.

After the match, Mr. Filiberto Emanuele came to my court #33 and played some tennis with me. He had excellent playing ability. This is no doubt helped by Mr. Tacchini as his tennis instructor.

After our playing, Mr. Emanuele gave me knighthood at a times 4 level. There was a royal photographer there to take pictures. I was informed that the Knighthood was official and recorded with the Kingdom of Italy.

After the Prince left the National Tennis Center in Flushing, NY. Vitas returned to talk to me about the visit. He told me the ATP office has officially recognized my Knighthood with their group. I was now cleared to play more tennis.

My pro tennis playing continued on court #33. As, I was ranked #4 and playing great. I was again asked to provide more backing to continue my tennis playing. This wasn't for Authority but for Sponsorship to play big pro tournaments. This also included the desire for the other pros to see me in newspaper and magazine articles. Before, Mr. Anthony Cambria, Mr. Patrick Mulrooney and Prince

Rackets were in charge of this. At first, I called my original sponsors but they couldn't help.

The next closest contact was Clemson University. I still had the admissions department phone number and they were happy to hear from me. They really liked the idea that I was on court #33 at the National Tennis Center. They are used to their students traveling to the tennis center to play tennis. They said "yes" they will back me playing at the National Tennis Center. I was finally making some progress.

To get more help, I then called some people I knew from where I grew up. One contact I knew was Sir. Richard Branson. I left a message with his front desk and later when I called back I was happy to find out he decided to sponsor my tennis at the National Tennis Center in Flushing, NY. This sponsorship helped me start to play more pro tournaments.

I knew Sir. Richard Branson from my neighborhood in Jericho, NY where the school district is connected to some exclusive areas. I had met him through one or more friends who knew him through their parents. I remember sometimes meeting him at 11:00 pm at night at my friend's house. He thought I could win big in life and gave me some advice. At that age, I remembered my schedule of staying up late and having to wake up early in the morning. After these meetings, I thought that my schedule must have been the path to success and wasn't just to wear me down.

My ranking soared above #4 and I was going to the rank of #1. This reality made it where my new sponsors gave me a phone call and told me they decided to build me my own tennis center at the Alley Pond Park, in Queens, NYC. The building of the Tennis Center took a few months to complete. It had a one-story clubhouse with a reception counter, glass panel viewing area, and a men's and women's locker room with bathrooms and showers. I even had my own $3,000 desk looking out at the tennis courts. The Tennis Center also had 6 hard surface tennis courts covered with a white tennis bubble. The bubble was supported with air pressure. The courts were well-lit for indoor playing. On the exterior, there was a nice entrance with a walkway. The tennis center had a large parking lot. This allowed everyone free parking in a big city setting.

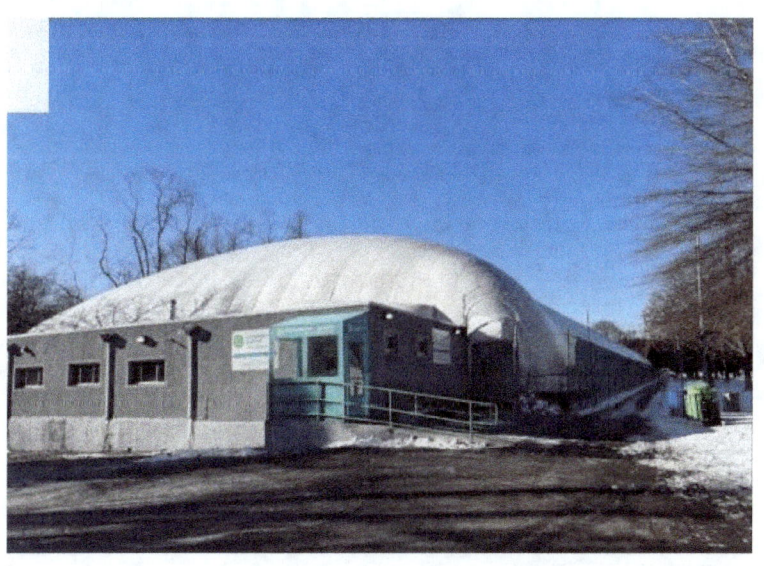

Photo: The Alley Pond Tennis Center.

This new reality that I am the top player made it were I would play at my tennis center some days of the week and other days at court #33. I started to hold 2 courts. As I started to play tennis at Alley Pond. The National Tennis Center started to send me players to teach. Since I was a top player and had great ability to win tournaments. The ATP administrators wanted me to teach the other-up-and-coming players. This idea wasn't new and I had taught some players in the past years. These tennis lessons I gave were very pricey. Some were between $10,000 and $15,000 per hour. The whole thing was set up with the National Tennis Center and the sponsors of the tennis players.

Some of the players I taught went on to win tournaments. They would come back for another lesson and tell me they just won a big tournament. Even though my students won tournaments they still couldn't beat me in a tennis match. I would always give them a chance to play me in a match at Alley Pond. This helped them to learn how to win.

At Alley Pond, there was a building Manager assigned to watch the facility and he helped with my tennis assignments. Henry was nice enough to bring me gifts of tennis hats, equipment, and desk supplies, etc. He would even take out his tennis racket and help me warm up in the morning. He would always hold up a glass of wine and give me a cheer when I won the match.

The other pro players coming to the National Tennis Center found their way over to the Alley Pond Tennis Center. One player that stopped in was Mr. Ken Rosewall. He was playing with the Australian team and was a veteran pro tennis player. Ken was friendly and we talked about tennis. He told me about the autobiography he wrote a few years earlier and asked that I read the book, so I could learn from his many years of pro tennis playing. In the days after that, I went to the local public library and withdrew the book. When Ken was at the Alley Pond Tennis Center again, I told him I read his book. Mr. Rosewall gave me a book quiz to see if I remembered what I had read. I answered all of his questions 100 percent correctly. Ken was so amazed that he glanced around the room and started to believe that this whole tennis center was made for me and I was reaching the top in pro tennis.

As I played at my Alley Pond Tennis Center there were some ideas of making the tennis center my own training center for learning where I would have paid classes with the general public. This would take some knowhow and even College education to unfold. But for now, the playing was just for pro tennis players. My sponsors were allowing the other pro players to use the facility when I wasn't there. As some wild behavior took place from visiting players. My sponsors were acting very open with the other pros. Our side realized if the tables were turned, they would ask for $10,000 an hour to enter. The building manager, Henry, was told to slowly tighten the entry requirements into the tennis center so they couldn't interfere with my playing.

One player that made it to my tennis center was Ms. Helena Sukova from Switzerland. She traveled to New York City to play the tournaments there with the other female pro players. In an unfortunate set of circumstances, she wasn't given any money after she arrived. Her situation came to my attention by the building manager, Henry. So, it was my decision to help Helena so she wouldn't go homeless. I decided to give her some money while she was staying in the USA. In the next few weeks and months, me and Helena made friends and she also started to tell me about her tennis playing. She was like a Cinderella story, playing top pro tennis as a female singles player. Helena had some smarts and as I played a series of Tournaments she would watch me play sitting at my desk. She was always cheering for me and giving me a big applause. On other occasions, she would get her tennis racket and help me warm-up before the match. I won a total of 15 tournaments at Alley Pond. Helena commented that she never saw anyone win that many pro tournaments, especially in a short time.

After a number of months, Ms. Helena Sukova had to leave the Alley Pond Tennis Center and return to Switzerland. Her stay had become exhausted and she needed to return home and recover from the misguided travel to the USA. After that, I was aware that she made more return trips to the USA without any problems. I further read years later that she continued her tennis career in Switzerland and became really successful.

One big tournament that took place at the National Tennis Center and Alley Pond was the Fischer Open. The final match was uncertain at the start of the tournament and it was played on different tennis courts. The player setup was similar to the 1987 US Open. The only difference is this tournament wasn't exclusionary.

I played the matches for the tournament like any other tournament. After a series of wins, I was told I made the final match for the Fischer Open by the building manager Henry. He told me I was to invite family and friends to attend this special event. It was scheduled in the evening so everyone could attend in person and it was also played live on ESPN and other television stations.

I invited my family, friends, and girlfriend Dahlia to attend the final match. I was confident to invite everybody. The special event was good for me and everyone I know. It was a big event at my new tennis center at Alley Pond, NYC.

The night of the final match the court was well prepared. The walls had Fischer signs around its borders with large Television cameras on stands. I used the locker room before the match started. My girlfriend Dahlia walked into the locker room and we talked before the match. She was happy to see this big event happen. It was something she had always hoped for. This is because we had talked many times about our future together with pro tennis and entertainment. The building manager Henry walked in and told us the event was starting. As we walked out together there were professional photographers and they took pictures of me and Dahlia together. Everyone could see us together as a couple in love.

When I was standing on the tennis court, I looked over at the glass panel wall and saw my sponsor Sir. Richard Branson with a group of friends. Behind them was my girlfriend Dahlia, including some of our common friends Heidi, Julie and Gina. To the left of my sponsors were my opponent's sponsors and some of his friends.

My opponent was Mr. Jonas Svensson from Sweden. He was 2 years older than me and had a tennis ranking of 10 or above. Certainly, he was a formidable opponent. He was already playing tennis matches at the National Tennis

Center for a long time. His sponsor was there in attendance behind the glass wall. She had traveled all the way from Sweden to watch the final tournament match.

I won the choice to serve and took that advantage. To start the match I pointed my tennis racket at the area in the opponent's serving box where I was going to serve the ball. The crowd started cheering for me. I hit the ball with a swift overhead serve. As I started winning the match my supporters and fans started cheering and giving me a lot of applause. I was able to play amazingly for this big match. I had a memorable crosscourt shot that made everyone act in awe. The match was mine, winning very confidently. That night I won the match and won the Fischer Open Tournament.

Afterwards, I had a trophy photograph session scheduled. I met Sir. Richard Branson and we had some photographs taken together with the trophy. Our all-day and all-night schedule was still going on and it was successful! This was a good time to talk to Richard about my tennis playing and he was really impressed and thought I was a big winner.

The next afternoon, my neighbor Mr. Hy Ozer walked out of his house when I was getting in my car. He congratulated me! Telling me he saw me win the tennis match on television. I told him about the Fischer Open and the tennis match. This confirmed people were seeing me win on television. It was exhilarating to get this feedback.

In pro tennis and any level tennis playing a particular tennis tournament might not be available to participate in. There are exclusive tournaments, clubs, etc. My sponsors were very honest and always participated in legal, honest and open tournaments.

When the fall of 1987 came the US Open wasn't on the list of fair and open tournaments. It had a reputation of "winning third place". The Captain of the pro players, Vitas, wanted me to play in the 1987 US Open. I said OK and I was told when to play. The players were the same ATP players I was used to playing in the tour. I won all five of the matches. This put me in the number 1 position in my group. The last match was on television against a different player from Sweden. He was in the Fischer Open but didn't make it to the final match. The US Open tennis match was really big. There were photographers holding big TV cameras. I won the match with-hundreds of attendees cheering and thousands of tennis fans watching me at home.

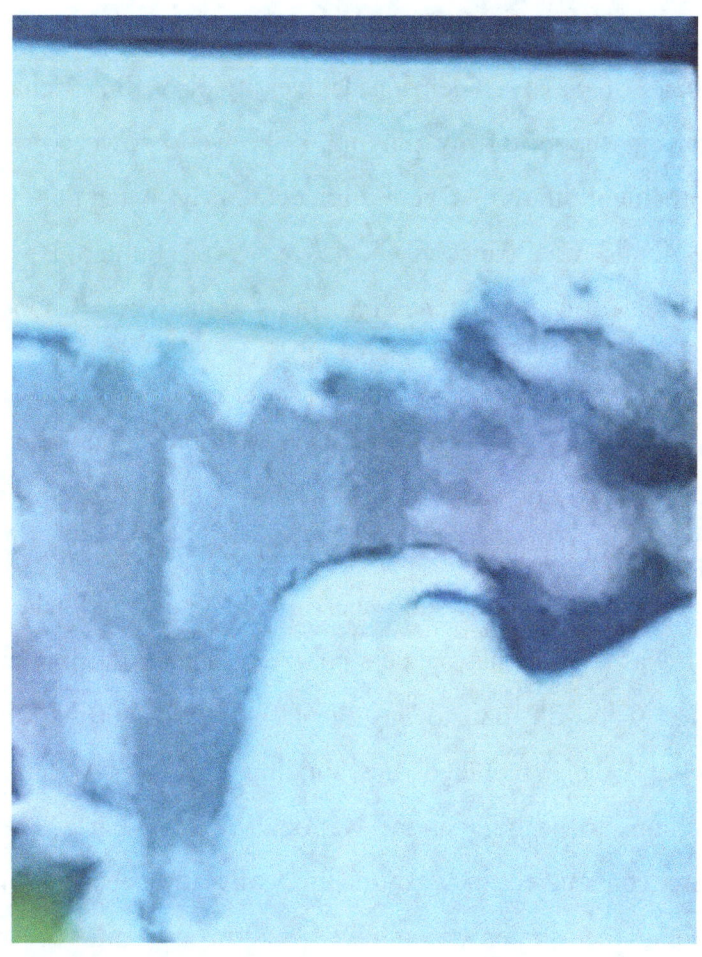

Photo: John Riggio at the National Tennis Center 1987.

I had told my girlfriend Dahlia about this US Open match and she really wanted to go. She paid admission to attend and found a seat courtside at the National Tennis Center. She had her admission ticket in her hand and my player name was written right on it, "John Rigo".

A big stop happened with this tournament. Even as the Prince of Savoy, Clemson University and Sir. Richard Branson supported my playing. The well-known corrupt tournament "the US Open" didn't care. My match date for the finals was canceled. This was even though I was undefeated in the matches up to this point. The US Open problem made a big quake take place with my sponsors.

Since the US Open didn't care about me, the number 1 player, they got sued in Court. This situation happened before with the US Open, when I was the number 1 ranked junior player. The lawsuit was so big no one would believe it. It wasn't in the newspapers but the settlement went in my favor. The ATP had to pay the USA nearly 400 Million Dollars. This included the funding for 3 new tennis stadiums to be built at the National Tennis Center. They were constructed in a short time after the decision. In theory, the agreement allowed me to use one of the stadiums. This would never unfold. They continued to resist my playing there.

The Australian team also had a watch on my tennis playing in the US Open that year. Since the tournament organizers didn't let me play though. The Australian team asked for permission to secure their own ranking numbers in Australia and left the USA a short time later.

On the cusp of further success, this new opportunity arose that would change everything. Striving past distractions that was like a funny movie that would make you laugh, and the cookery around me, that would make you cry. My new sponsors instantly put the past behind me and boosted my career. I was successful to have maneuvered through official channels and secured this new great future.

My tennis playing at this point was starting to generate a lot of money in pro tennis. The value of my contract zoomed up from $500,000 to 5 Million US Dollars and was ready to move up even further. From my obvious great value in the sports business, my contract was sold. Sir. Branson sold my tennis contract to Ms. Gloria Vanderbilt and company for a staggering 5 Million US Dollars.

Chapter Five
Playing in Manhattan

The previous tennis center in Alley Pond was left behind. The New York City Parks Department leased the building and courts to some tennis instructors. It continued to grow and ultimately became the largest tennis bubble in the whole United States of America.

My new tennis center was constructed at Sutton East, Manhattan, NYC. At the corner of East 59th Street between York Avenue and Sutton Place, Manhattan, NY. Some pieces of my previous tennis center were relocated. This included the white tennis bubble and the wall of pane-glass. The overall structure of the main bubble was very large. It could house 3 or more 5-court tennis bubbles inside its structure. The outside cover of this sports complex is the largest bubble in all of the Borough of Manhattan, NYC. There was a new entrance constructed on Sutton Place with glass doors that open into a lobby area. On the left side I had my own locker and bathroom with my own entrance door onto the tennis courts. Straight ahead were the pane glass windows for clear viewing into the courts. To the right side was the glassed in sponsor area with a front desk for the building manager. The building manager was named Bill, he was only working for my new tennis center. He replaced the slot that Henry had at the Alley Pond Tennis Center.

On the first day of playing at the Sutton East Tennis Center I was greeted by my new sponsor Ms. Gloria Vanderbilt. She introduced herself and told me how the organizational structure of the sponsorship was going to proceed. Her whole personal situation with her family was also divulged. This was the first sponsor to express these things to me. I was able to get a whole picture of my new sponsor. Ms. Vanderbilt was a devout church goer and was always striving to do the correct things in life. This made me feel more relaxed and reassured me I was with good people and strong too. When I was playing tennis at the Sutton East Tennis Center, Ms. Vanderbilt always asked for my input. Even from the first day there I always gave her valuable replies to her questions.

When Ms. Gloria Vanderbilt wasn't talking directly to me, the building manager Bill would tell me my playing schedule. He would forward over to me what was happening with my sponsors.

To get the playing started the owner of the main Tennis bubble Mr. Tony Scolnick was my official tennis Administrator for pro tennis playing. His role was similar to Mr. Anthony Cambria. Mr. Scolnick was well-educated in sport management. With a doctor's degree in Physical Education. Mr. Scolnick knew how I could start playing matches real quick. To sharpen my tennis game at Sutton East, I started with players he had available. I then moved up to his tournament matches. After I was ready, I started to play the pro tour again. This warmup of games was excellently put together.

Ms. Gloria Vanderbilt's investment might have seemed like a huge amount of money that could not unfold. This wasn't the case. My playing ability was so steady that in just two weeks into my playing, she profited immensely. This covered all of the contract price multiplied by ten. Even the yearly lease for the Sutton East Tennis Center was paid off.

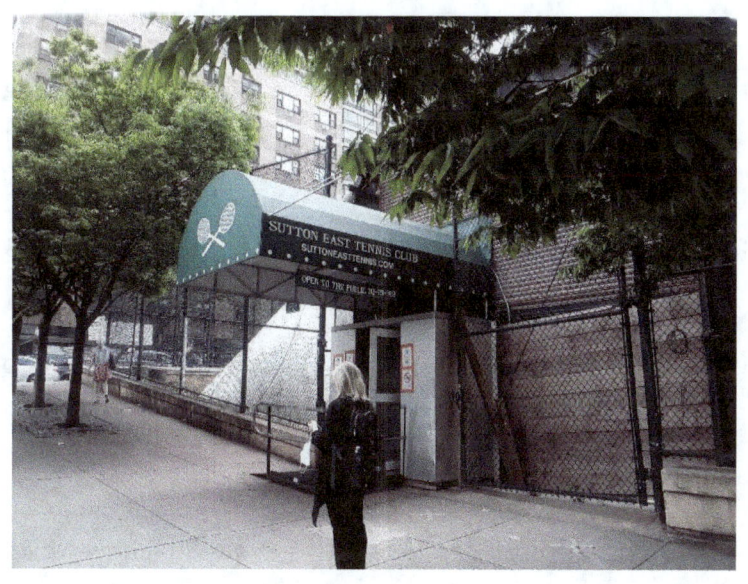

Photo: Entrance to the Sutton East Tennis Center.

The pro tournament playing continued. I was holding my own court by winning matches and tournaments. This started to take the usual pattern of a new sponsor. As the tournament started, I was talking to Ms. Vanderbilt and she told me I needed a new player name. My previous name "John Rigo" is over and my new tennis name must start. She got on the telephone with the ATP office and proposed some new names. Gloria asked me what name I wanted. I said "John East". This is from the street sign East 59th Street. The name was forwarded instantly. The male ATP office worker said "No". We were out of names. He persuaded Ms. Vanderbilt to use "John Vanderbilt".

The use of this name became much bigger in writing than usual. Gloria was working hard at making me a big name in tennis. She started with an advertisement in one of the Manhattan publications. It was an autograph signing invitation to get fans involved and add to my playing career. The advertisement and the autograph signing went great. Many people young and old arrived at the Sutton East Tennis Center and I talked to them and signed autographs. They were very happy to see me.

The next pro player add-on was to have a tennis racket brand as a sponsor. Ms. Vanderbilt told me Slazenger Rackets are willing to sponsor me. The previous company Prince Racket was gone with the contract sale. Slazenger sent a representative to the Sutton East Tennis Center. The building manager gave me sweats, two Slazenger tennis rackets and a bag. I also received some stickers. Slazenger also set up a photography session for me. The courts were set up with wall signage and their banner on the net. Their photographer arrived at the Sutton East Tennis Center and took a series of photos of me hitting the tennis ball with the Slazenger brand racket while wearing the Slazenger sweatsuit. I moved around the court showing him some of my different tennis shots as the photos were taken.

The next thing was to try out the Slazenger Tennis rackets in a match. As I played with Slazengers newest tennis racket the frame started to bend. I had to switch back to my pro stock racket I received from Mr. Patrick Mulrooney.

I returned the rackets to the building manager Bill. He ended up giving the rackets to Courtney. Courtney was a female pro tennis player. Since men and women pro players stay apart most of the time. Courtney was selected to play tennis as my counterpart. Her courts were on the other side of the main bubble. This is the area for the general public. Just by chance, I was there when she brought the two rackets back. They realized I bent two rackets in my last tennis match. Courtney was so amazed how each racket had a bent frame that she kept them for herself and bought two new tennis rackets to replace them.

At the Sutton East Tennis Center, Courtney came to my court and we played a tennis match. She was an excellent player and was highly ranked amongst the female pros. Courtney told me she was able to win against some male players. My winning streak against female players continued and she couldn't overtake me. I won the match. We finished by hitting the ball. She was a very nice counterpart to my sponsorship and a friend in our tennis struggles.

The new sponsor Ms. Gloria Vanderbilt also comprised different investors. This is typical in the sports business. Gloria created a corporation for her sports business. One person involved with my new sponsor was Mr. Robert Kraft. He was very experienced in tennis. He already owned a tennis franchise in the World Team Tennis League and sold it. At the time Mr. Kraft was just starting a new venture to own the American football team the New England Patriots.

I talked to Mr. Kraft and learned about tennis playing and sports business. Mr. Kraft watched a lot of my matches and saw me win some big tournaments at Sutton East. My contract expired with the ATP in the middle of the tournament season. Mr. Robert Kraft had the knowhow to apply for my contract to continue on. In the long wait. He made business papers to form a new pro tennis league. I started playing in the league right away. My opponents were the same as the ATP. These were the very best players and they were very happy about the new league. The ATP was very imperfect and the other players encountered the same problems.

The ATP approached Mr. Robert Kraft about the new tennis league he made. From these discussions, Mr. Kraft's new tennis league was bought by the ATP. The long-term value of the new league was lost. The only short-term success was that I wasn't stopped from playing pro tennis.

Mr. Kraft was very timely and helped with providing ESPN to my matches. He also helped with some TV interviews. The TV audience could watch me talk about my tennis matches after they were finished. Robert became very excited about my winning matches and tournaments. He always told me I could win big in sports.

This was also the time when I formulated my own tennis-playing strategy. This strategy also fulfilled the request of Mr. Tony Roche of Australia. Making my own tennis playing strategy topped off my tennis abilities. My winning percentage edged up to where I was close to unstoppable. From this new improvement, Mr. Robert Kraft gave me a big round of applause.

The idea of more and more spectators and a bigger TV audience grew. It grew to a point where Ms. Vanderbilt and Mr. Kraft worked on ideas to solve this need. The idea of building a grandstand for paid spectators was the new plan. This idea was successful. Gloria hired a designer from

Europe and a contractor. The stylish design of red seats and a glass handrail were constructed next to my bubble. It came with a giant flat screen TV.

My sponsors at Sutton East Tennis Center were filling in every item in the pro playing handbook. As I played tennis, a following of fans started to fill the tennis center lobby. One fan from South Korea used to come there on a daily basis and watched my matches. She used to wear very tight clothes and even brought her small pet dog. We used to talk in between matches and started to get to know each other. She liked my tennis playing so much she spread the word of my playing to her friends. She liked my natural name the best and didn't care about player names.

There were many fans walking in and out of the tennis center front doors. As I talked to these spectators in the lobby, many turned out to be well-known entertainers.

Some new fans I met in the lobby was Mr. Jaime Spears and next to him was his daughter Ms. Brittney Spears. After some weeks of seeing me play, Mr. Spears calculated my tennis contract value at $25 Million Dollars. Jaime invited me to play on the Hermon Park Tennis Courts located in Los Angeles, California. I did eventually visit the courts he suggested just a short time later. With this new friendship with Jaime Spears came a new introduction with his daughter Ms. Brittney Spears. She already had a music entertainment career and was well known. Brittney was a regular visitor to the Sutton East Tennis Center. We became good friends and we started to talk in the lobby of the tennis center and on the telephone after hours. I eventually met some more of her family and friends. Mr. Sam Asghari was always cheering my tennis career and was a common friend of the Spears family. When he used to visit the Sutton East Tennis Center we always talked as friends.

Before and after I won a big match at the Sutton East Tennis Center, I would get flooded with fans. My fans were so excited and would always greet me as I exited the tennis courts. Some of my new fans would stay around the lobby awhile and talk with me. This went on for months. I knew their names and we started to make friends. A lot of them had entertainment careers of their own.

One of my most devoted fans and friends was Liz. Who moved to NYC and was living in the area. She frequently snuck in to see me whenever she had free time from her entertainment aspirations. We talked together and got to know each other pretty well.

Some other entertainers I was introduced to who are big names in entertainment were Ms. Lisa Marie Presley, Jon Bon Jovi, Chuck Norris and Jackie Chan.

With playing long hours at the Sutton East Tennis Center came new abilities I developed. This was the amazing ability to sleep while standing up. While playing on the court I wasn't allowed to leave unless my matches were finished for the afternoon, or basic things like going to the bathroom or walking outside to have something to eat and drink. The time gap between each match was five minutes to one hour. If I didn't need to leave the courts I would start to just rest. This rest time would turn into a nap if it was longer than a few minutes. When the next opponent finally showed up I would reawaken and get ready to play.

The next benefit of my playing was a fancy sports car. I visited the car showroom in Manhattan and talked to the Salesman. There was a room filled with exotic cars like you would see in the movies. The Mercedes Benz car had a very expensive $50,000 lease and was to stay parked in front of the Sutton East Tennis Center for 6 months. It was a symbol of my successful pro tennis playing. The rich and sporty look matched the money and greatness I was creating on the tennis court.

The tournaments I won at Sutton East Tennis Center are the best in the world. One tournament that made a big milestone in my career was winning the Manhattan Open. This tournament was always bigger and better than the US Open. I have inserted an excerpt of the tournament levels. There is a full chart of pro matches in the back of this book.

Tennis Tournament Levels

1.American Airlines, Manhattan Open, Eastern Tournament, London Queens, Paris-Bercy, Lisbon, Portugal, Roland Garros

Other ATP tournaments: **Chicago, Illinois, Nashville, Tennessee, Dallas, Texas, Miami, Florida**

2.US Open, Laver Cup, French Open, Wimbledon
Other ATP tournaments: **ABN**
ATP Starter tournaments - **Vienne**

Before the tournament started I stopped back at the National Tennis Center in Flushing, NY. I was there for a required check-in to keep my ranking current. I talked to one of the players in charge and he told me I can continue playing at Sutton East, there is no need for a checkup. As he stood there with some other pro players he said. "Hey John, we are going to play the Manhattan Open this year. We will see you in the tournament matches." From this I understood they were going to play some tournaments I am involved with. Instead of being centered on the US Open. I knew I was allowed to play an honest game with my sponsors.

The Manhattan Open matches started. I was told by my sponsors that the player ranking of the Manhattan Open turns out to be 250 player rankings higher than the US Open. I played the matches in the tournament very competitively. I made the final match and it was at the Sutton East Tennis Center. That puts me 250 players higher than the US Open.

The final for the Manhattan Open arrived and there was a lot of preparation for the match. The ESPN cameras were in place. There was a viewing area filled with spectators. Even the blocks around the event were full of spectators.

I played the match with full confidence. With years of experience playing pro finals, I was able to handle this level of playing. I had to focus my mind on winning.

Giving that extra effort to surpass my opponent in each game of the set. I met the challenge and won the match and the Manhattan Open.

My opponent left first and was given his 2nd place prize. After this, I exited to the lobby of the tennis center. There I was greeted by my fans. They were cheering, grabbing me and kissing me. I looked outside and saw the street filled with people cheering. Ms. Gloria Vanderbilt walked over and congratulated me. There was a very large trophy presented to me. Photographers were present taking pictures of me with Gloria and the Trophy. There were even pictures taken of me kissing the Trophy. It was a great night!

This tournament made me a special part of New York City. It was suggested that I live in New York City to benefit from my great victory. I was to later find out this tournament is world famous and everyone watches it on world television.

Another tournament I won that was very big was the Eastern Tournament. This was a great tournament. The Eastern was a tournament of many matches. It took a long time to rise to the final and win. I had the same feeling when I won the Eastern tournament as a junior.

The American Airlines Open was another big tournament and there was a big final match at Sutton East. The spectators were cheering in the grandstand and in the lobby. This tournament was internationally televised on ESPN. This was a memorable tournament. It is considered one of the best in the USA.

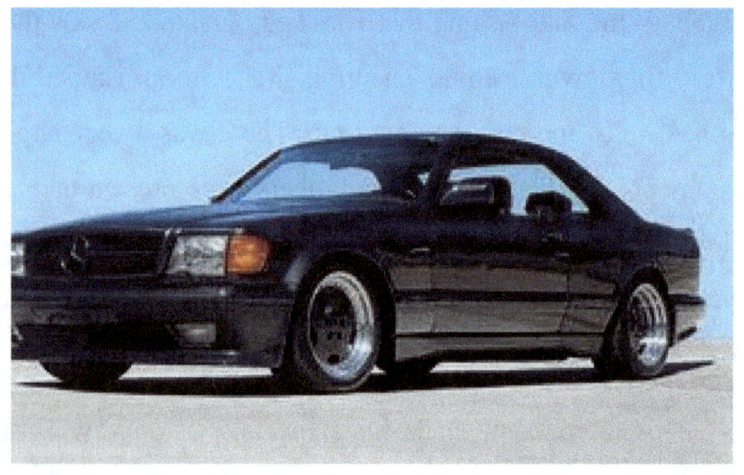

Photo: 1990 Mercedes Benz at Sutton East Tennis Center.

The tournaments at the Sutton East Tennis Center were also international. Since I was the number 1 player, I still held my own court. In the ATP there were some international tournaments available like the London Queens, Paris Bercy, Lisbon, Portugal. These were excellent tournaments and I won the international title in each one. This included a Trophy and Certificate showing that I won. All of these priceless items are held by my sponsors. With each tournament win there was the opportunity to live in each country and play tennis. Each country offered advertising that I won big if I stayed there a certain number of years. Some requested me to live in their country for a number of years to reap the benefits of glory.

A memorable international tournament was called the Lisbon Portugal. I played with all of the tennis players from Portugal. The Portugal team claimed they were the best pro tennis players in the world. As I played the portugal tournament I played the portugal team and many pro players that were signed up to play the Lisbon tournament. They were also some of the best players in the world. I started to play the tournament and was on my usual winning streak in the tournament. I played one opponent that was from Portugal. He was able to win the match. He wasn't their highest ranked player and that gave me a chance at playing him a second time. Before the match he admitted that I was the number one player in the world. He was exclaiming that he could become the number one ranked player. I told him winning one match doesn't make you the number one player so fast. He didn't care and felt the importance of this match to advance. After losing one match to him reset the scorecard for me, I could now start winning another group of matches. We played the match. The excitement the player from Portugal brought with him was very good. I stayed as sharp as possible and concentrated real hard at winning each point. He played very well, but after reviewing his previous match in my mind I was able to maximize the winning shots and minimize the losing shots. I also looked to keep on the offensive, and not let my game become defensive. With all of these playing skills coming together I won the match with full confidence.

I was to win the Lisbon Portugal tournament on the International track. This is the highest track and is where all of the monetary prizes are from. To get local recognition in Portugal, I would have to live there for nine years. I turned down that offer and instead my sponsors received the trophy and certificate for my International play.

One international tournament I was number 1 placed to win was the Roland Garros in Spain. That particular tournament required the players to attend in Spain for the final match. Since me and my sponsors were busy at the Sutton East Tennis Center we didn't attend.

With each international tournament, there were many players from around the world. Over the years I was always playing people from around the world through the ATP and the National Tennis Center. These players were the same but were more visible as star players when they came to play a match at the Sutton East Tennis Center. The groups of players were clearly visible. Some groups were from Britain, Portugal, Spain, France, Sweden, Australia, and Argentina.

I was playing the pro tour with some excellent players. One of the players was Mr. Luis Madero. He had played me a few times before, starting all the way back in 1985 at my courts in Jericho, NY. He was usually with a group of players from Argentina and Spain. When we played at the Sutton East Tennis Center he won a match. I did lose a few matches of tennis, but not that many. Since he won one match, my sponsors wanted to see if Luis had the skills to win against me and had him play me several times. Mr. Luis Madero was willing to play these additional matches. This also gave me time to figure out how to win the match myself. I always tried to think about how my opponent played the ball, what his passing shots were. I noticed Luis had a drop shot to my left side that was getting him the extra points he needed to win the match. I would have to find a new shot to get the ball past them in a game. I started to work on a new tennis shot to patch the hole in my game that Luis had exploited. I did find a new shot, it was a sweeping hit of the ball where I would give the ball such a high spin that the ball would go right down the right side of his court. It was too fast for him to swing and hit the ball back. We played another match at the Sutton East Tennis Center. The game was well played, Luis was a very experienced tennis player. Then Luis tried placing his winning shot past me to my left side. I ran back in position and made my sweep of the tennis ball. The ball quickly passed his right side, just as I had practiced. He couldn't even get close to the ball. As we played the rest of the match he tried a few times to make his winning shot again but I kept giving him a sweep of the ball right past him. I won the match. Since Mr. Luis Madero played an exciting match, my sponsors had him return a few more times to play additional matches against me. He wasn't able to win another match. At the end of the last match we played, he was very impressed and we talked about pro tennis. I gave him a quick lesson on my tennis playing skills. He could always use these in his next match. I wasn't afraid to give away some playing secrets.

Another memorable tournament was the London Queens. This was a tournament that was televised in the United States of America. Many people watch the matches and recognize the tournament name. The tournament also had many top players from around the world that participated. I was able to play all of the players from Britain. This included their number one team member and highest ranked player. He was a young player, about the same age as myself. We had an excellent match. It was a hard and competitive set of games. I had to use all of my usual concentration and repertoire of shots to win the match. This kind of effort to win this match was typical in all of the matches I played in the tournament. In total I won all of the matches of the tournament. I was playing through my usual winning streak. One match was against the well-known player Mr. John Llyod from Britain. We talked together and had a friendly conversation. He was a veteran player and was used to frequenting New York City. Playing their team and this tournament went very well in person. There wasn't any cheating or complaints that they wanted to win the match. In all I won the London Queens-International. My sponsors received a large trophy and certificate. To win on the domestic track would involve my living in Britain for 3 to 6 years. I was forwarded this offer through my sponsors but I turned it down. There was too much uncertainty that leaving the USA would really give me any more attention for this tournament that I already received.

The brand new Grandstand exceeded its expected success in just a short time. The large crowds of spectators gathered around the tennis center and sat on the grandstand to view my matches shown on the Flat Panel screen. The city observed the overflowing crowds and started to question the tennis center's capacity for that mass of spectators. The Sutton East Tennis Center and its encompassing structure is part of the New York City Public property. The City made an internal inspection and put in writing for the tennis center to make changes for the overflow of the excessive spectators. The NYC DOB gave the Sutton East Tennis Center a deadline to comply. There were some studies made of the tennis center trying to keep the Grandstand, but it wasn't feasible.

My sponsors sold the Grandstand to the Times Square Development company. The designer who prepared the original drawings for the grandstand did excellent work. The value of the Grandstand continued on and is now located in Times Square Manhattan, NYC. It was renovated years later, but kept the same look of red seating and glass.

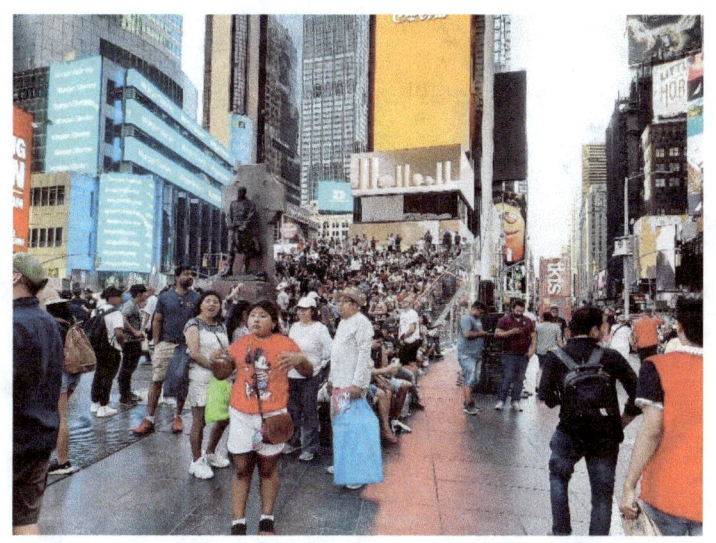

Photo: My relocated Grandstand in Times Square Manhattan, NYC.

The next answer to keep the crowds going at my tennis matches was to build a new tennis stadium. Ms. Gloria Vanderbilt acted very quickly to have design and construction drawings made. The funding part was worked out with her partners in my sponsorship. Even the stadium's name was formed. It wasn't named after me. It was named after the loan financier "Chase Bank". A location was found in the old polo grounds of Manhattan, NYC. There were stadiums built long ago for playing polo and baseball.

Soon after, I saw Gloria with a big set of construction drawings in the office at Sutton East. Everything was ok with the plans and permits and construction started. Some work on the site has begun.

The only thing about the Stadium is that tennis isn't considered a stadium sport. The pier pressure to construct a stadium instead of a better tennis center with a grandstand was a problem. Around the National Tennis Center, most people think tennis is jealous of Baseball. They had the big Shea Stadium with the NY Mets next door. I was hoping this stadium idea would work out.

One morning I arrived at the Sutton East Tennis Center and the doors were locked and there was a sign.stating the tennis center was closed indefinitely. I returned back home. I called the manager's office a number of times but there was no answer. Finally I received a phone call from the building manager, Bill. He told me the unfortunate news of the death of Ms. Gloria Vanderbilt's son Mr. Carter Cooper. He died one day near his home, I was never told the details. Bill explained Gloria was mourning the death of her son. I was asked to wait for a phone call about my tennis playing status.

The tennis world was both fierce and rewarding, but I was ever prepared to embrace the thrill of competition, to forge unbreakable bonds, and to claim my rightful place in the annals of professional tennis. As I continued to improve and gain recognition, the future sparkled with the potential of what lay ahead.

Chapter Six
On the Road and Back

The closed Sutton East Tennis Center left me wondering if the tennis playing is over with this sponsor. The death of Ms. Gloria Vanderbilt's son Mr. Carter Cooper was in all of the newspapers and seen on the television news. The grief of this horrible event seemed to last a long time. Even today they still have news, books and videos about the death of Mr. Carter Cooper.

In previous years at the Sutton East Tennis Center, I used to talk to Mr. Carter Cooper. He was just a few years older than me. He was the older and only brother to Mr. Andersen Cooper. Carter and I played a match of tennis together on my court. He was competitive in spirit. As we played he started to believe I was a great pro player. My great tennis playing won the fun match and he gained first-hand knowledge of my playing skills.

When Carter Cooper was watching my tennis matches there were a lot of fans and friends of the sponsors present. They all assembled in the lobby of the Sutton East Tennis

Center. Everyone was making new friends. It became a social event with my pro tennis playing as the main subject. This group of people loved my run of playing tournaments. They were all rallying around the profits and victories of my playing. Everyone was also young and learning about sports and entertainment. There was a comfortable atmosphere in the room, like a pro version of a home BBQ party.

From my fan club came a big surprise. I received a phone call from someone who was friends with the sponsors. Since my fans loved my playing so much he told me they made him the Representative to have me continue pro tennis playing. He said he would call with a time, date and location to play the next tennis match. This was good, because I didn't have to wait before I could restart my tennis-playing abilities.

The new sponsor Representative was able to connect with the National Tennis Center and have pro matches arranged. The only difference with this continuation of my playing was there was no Sutton East Tennis Center to play at. I then started to play at different court locations. The playing was just some pro players they had available. I was able to win my matches as usual.

The new Rep. did excellent work. He had a video camera with him and always acted like a coach watching each game from start to finish. This arrangement could take me anywhere in the world. It was something different than having my own court all of the time.

This new venture showed there was no magic in having my own court. My opponents couldn't win against me. I could handle driving to a tennis match and still play great. They also couldn't get away with cheating. The new leader had the video and knew who to call in the ATP.

There was one memorable tennis match I played at this time. The new sponsor Representative arranged an ATP match located in the Borough of Queens, inside New York City. I drove to the outdoor courts and met my sponsor Rep. and my opponent. The opponent had a coach with him on court side to watch the tennis match. The match was videotaped by my sponsor. I had played this opponent years earlier and it was good to play again. I know from the first meeting he probably wanted to make a deal with me taking the fall. I don't make deals, they are bad for my tennis career and could be dangerous. My opponent's player ranking was low in real terms but he was much higher ranked in the magazines. As we played the match, I was very confident and used all of my tennis skills to play an excellent game. He admitted I was playing great and started to get tired during the match, he didn't even want to finish the match. It was a big romp and I won the match very quickly. He wasn't so happy about losing and started to act unsportsmanlike. After losing the match he just left the courts in a hurry with his coach. My sponsor Rep. was there and gave me a big round of applause.

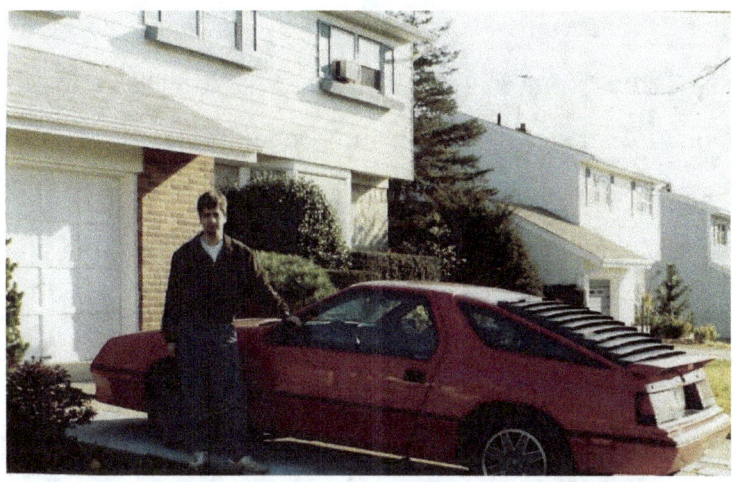

Photo: John Riggio standing next to his car at home in Jericho, NY 1990.

Months passed as I played pro tennis for my fan club. I was getting very impressed with the sponsor Rep., this situation could have me tour anywhere. My winning percentage was still the same. The Rep. knew all of the things to cover sponsoring my matches. The opponents they sent from the ATP couldn't cheat and lie. This traveling situation could get me to different locations that required I visit their courts. For example, one tournament that required an in person visit to play the finals was the Roland Garros. The Davis Cup, also required an in person visit.

One afternoon, I received a phone call from Ms. Gloria Vanderbilt. I hadn't talked to her since the Sutton East Tennis Center closed their doors. When answering the phone I immediately gave her my condolences about Carter Cooper. She was of course still in mourning for her son and told me that she received a phone call about my fan club playing me in the ATP.

My fan club members were still relying on Gloria and the Sutton East Tennis Center as the main sponsor. They were officially business associates. From the love of my fans Gloria put her problems aside and decided to continue my pro tennis playing at the Sutton East Tennis Center.

The next week the closed sign was removed from the tennis center doors and I was back on my court. The tournament matches started again. I was back winning. Gloria decided to restart some perks they gave me. One was a new autograph signing at the Sutton East Tennis Center.

Ms. Vanderbilt also was applying for me to obtain the award of ATP player of the year. I did receive the ATP Most Valuable Player of the year award that year. I have received other ATP awards over the past years and have some all time ATP records.

As my pro tennis playing continued, I won the prestigious tournament the American Airlines Open. All of my fans were cheering in the lobby of the tennis center and the final match was seen on national and international television. The trophy was brought out to me for some photographs. This was a great tournament to win.

This stimulated the ATP to send one of their representatives to talk to Ms. Gloria Vanderbilt and me. I talked to this lady in the lobby of the Sutton East Tennis Center. She was about 30 years old. She congratulated me for winning the big tournament. She hoped I would have many more years of playing.

She was very nice to me but when she talked to Ms. Gloria Vanderbilt was a double-crosser. The ATP employee threatened to kill Ms. Vanderbilt. Gloria knew how to handle this kind of problem and called the NYC Police Department.

The ATP employee was arrested and convicted of a crime. She went to prison and was let out a short time later. At the tennis center, the ATP employee also told a tale of getting Millions of Dollars a year from the pro player fees and spending it wildly. Since she always got away with these crimes she would tell everyone she was a "God".

The problems with this ATP employee didn't just stop with her getting sent to jail. After she was released the ATP employee returned to the Sutton East Tennis Center with a gun to find my sponsors. This ATP employee was unaware that Gloria had her own security guards. The bodyguards were able to grab the ATP employee and call the Police. The Police arrested the employee and she was charged with attempted murder.

This was never big in the local New York City newspapers, but there was a criminal court case shortly after with Ms. Gloria Vanderbilt, the plaintiff and the ATP employee, the defendant. The ATP lady was convicted to 5 years in prison. She did go to jail to serve her sentence. A few months later, I was told the ATP employee had died in prison.

As this happened my playing continued on. I was still winning a lot of matches and tournaments. My playing percentage was still at an unbelievable level. I had runs of winning 40 matches in a row. The details of my playing on the court were getting better and better. I usually would hit the ball over the net 25 times in a row without it going out.

There were a lot of tournaments to play. Some were Chicago, Illinois, Nashville, Tennessee, Dallas, Texas, Miami, Florida. These were all top tournaments. Higher than the US Open.

In one tournament, the Chicago Open, I played Mr. Guillermo Vilas. He was a veteran player of more than 16 years my senior and was the favorite to win the tournament. I already knew him and had played matches against him before. He was a friendly contestant. This is because he was a real winner.

We played the match and I won. I didn't think I would lose because of my steady playing. This wasn't the final match of the tournament. I played another pro vying to win and in the final match, I played past him and won. I won the match and the Chicago Open.

As a big promotional effort to advertise my tennis playing career. My sponsors requested a Slazenger tennis racket to have my player name printed on it and have it sold in stores. This wish was granted and the racket was found on the stores shelves in the Midwest of the United States of America. Gloria bought one of the rackets and she had it laying on the desk of her office. I saw proof of the racket myself, looking from the lobby of the Sutton East Tennis Center. Since I wasn't keeping a scrapbook, I didn't buy my own copy of the tennis racket. This is just another piece of my tennis history to think about.

Ms. Vanderbilt wanted me to grow big in life and expand as a pro tennis player. She had asked me about my travels and I told her how I did visit many cities with my father and mother by automobile. My father even drove our whole family in his new Chevrolet from Long Island New York to California and back. Of course, I recounted my vacation trip to Puerto Rico as part of my contract signing with Anthony Cambria. I was still in College and living with my family. Gloria called my mother, Rose, and asked her to have me take some travel vacations so I can see the world. This was also to have fun with some tennis playing around the world. My mother agreed to this idea and during the summer we took a two week vacation package to Italy. It was a very nice tour with 4 and 5 star hotels. On the tour through Italy, I made a new friend, Josephine, who was traveling with us in a group. When we walked together in Rome the Paparazzi started to walk over and took photographs of us together. Wondering why someone was taking pictures so directly and in an excited hurry, I told her about my pro tennis playing. On one occasion an interested group was there taking photographs of me. As I waved to the crowd they replied with great applause. I was eager to return back and continue my tournament run.

The dangers of pro tennis weren't just for my sponsors. At one tournament that I won. There was a crowd of one hundred people or more in the Sutton East Tennis Center lobby and hundreds of people outside the door on the sidewalk and street. They were all there to greet me and celebrate my big tournament victory. As I stood there in front of the crowd, I shook hands and gave hugs. All of a sudden a male spectator about the same age and height as myself approached. He started to squeeze between two of my fans. In a few seconds he lunged at me with a knife. I quickly punched him in the nose and knocked him out. Everyone was in awe. When someone yelled "look the attacker's knife is on the floor!" a lot of people started screaming. My sponsors took care of the rest by calling the Police Department.

I usually have my girlfriend Dahlia come to my matches. While playing at Sutton East Tennis Center I was still meeting Dahlia and telling her about my pro tennis. The Sutton East Tennis Center was in the Borough of Manhattan, NYC and she didn't want to visit. It wasn't me, otherwise it was Manhattan, NYC she thought was too overwhelming with potential dangers to venture there. The same was for some of my other common friends with Dahlia. So they could only hear the stories and watch the matches on television.

Some amazing things started to develop at the Sutton East Tennis Center. One was that the players that traveled to Manhattan, NYC could stay in an apartment adjacent to the south side of the Tennis Bubble. This idea worked very well and at the time of the match, my opponent would just walk across the street and enter the tennis center.

Even with making these amenities, there were other problems with some of the other pro players. My tennis playing was so great that the usual jealousy developed. The anger of some of my opponents started to manifest themselves into a desire to kill me.

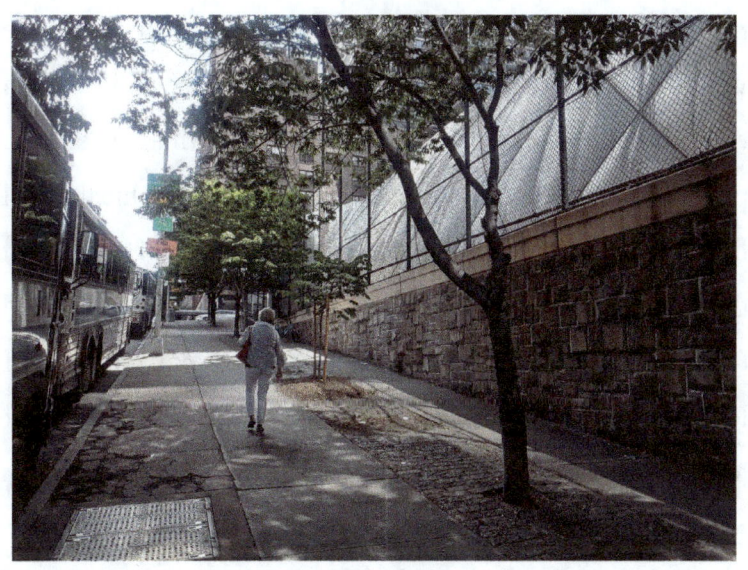

Photo: South Side of the Sutton East Tennis Center.

My sponsors were given some death threats against me. The building manager Bill told me about this and said my sponsors had a plan to keep me safe as I left the Sutton East Tennis Center each night. After a tennis match, Bill would find my opponent and watch him visually. I was then told to walk to my car by one of the staff members. This worked very well and I didn't have any problems getting harmed.

In one big final match of a tournament at Sutton East Tennis Center was played by my old student from Alley Pond Tennis Center. He was an up-and-coming pro that the National Tennis Center wanted me to teach. I always taught players how to win matches. The game was very hard. He was still playing pro and winning. The game didn't seem right. His ball hitting was way past the normal speed of a pro tennis racket. I could see him lean back to hit the ball like it was a heavy object. Most players lean forward to hit the ball. It looked like he won the final match and tournament. He was happy and started to exit the court. I looked down and was sad to lose the match. I almost never lose a tournament final match.

Then I see my sponsor come over to meet my opponent. This is usually to thank him for playing. My sponsor instead inspected his tennis racket and the racket proved to be illegal. My former student had bought a racket from someone at the National Tennis Center and it was contraband. This is an illegally made tennis racket that is strung to 73 lbs and weights 14 oz. The usual tennis racket is strung to 60 lbs to 65 lbs max with a common racket weight of 10.7 oz to 11.3 oz.

The final match was canceled from the record. The ATP was very light on my former student with the illegal tennis racket. The ATP decided that I play a rematch with my opponent using a regulation tennis racket. The rematch took place at Sutton East Tennis Center. I played the match as usual. My opponent was noticeably using a legal racket. The heavy and high-strung illegal tennis racket was set aside. I easily won the match. Ms. Gloria Vanderbilt received the Trophy and the Certificate of proof.

Additionally, the issue of illegal equipment loomed large in this environment of deceit. I learned that some players were utilizing racket designs that exceeded standard dimensions, giving them an unfair competitive edge. These rackets, constructed through dubious means and disguised to appear as legitimate brands, often had altered weights and string tensions that could significantly impact play. I came across one player who proudly displayed a racket that was noticeably heavier than the regulation limit. This increasing occurrence of my opponents using illegal tennis rackets was the reason why a pro shop was required. Each tennis racket is required to get documented in the owner's books and kept on file for verification if necessary. Since all of my rackets were given to me by Mr. Patrick Mulrooney of S&S sports, I was safe using only legally documented tennis rackets and strung within the legal tension amounts. The off the shelf rackets handed to me by Prince and Slazenger were also a legal standard.

My tennis player name John Vanderbilt was a good strong name. Even though a lot of people liked the name, There were some fundamental problems with the name John Vanderbilt. One was that it was forced on us by the ATP office. This was similar to when the ATP forced me to use the name John Holton when I was still a Junior player. Another reason is that it isn't allowed to use the name Vanderbilt. It is one of a few special names that the United States of America doesn't want duplicated. This is because many people are scammers trying to get money out of people's families and just by using their last name.

The next problem was everyone liked my natural name Mr. John Riggio. As time went on at the Sutton East Tennis Center everyone knew me as John Riggio. The player name was only used with some people. I was always very sensitive to people who like the name John Vanderbilt. I was used to having a player name.

The player name problem started to boil up again. There was Mr. Sam Asghari who was my sponsor's friend and frequent spectator of my tennis matches. He started to speak up about my new tennis playing card that was just published. It had my photograph and said Top Pro Player. The name was John Vanderbilt.

The new idea was to mirror my career with my natural name. Mr. Sam Asghari talked to Gloria and asked to have my pro tennis trading card made with my natural name. She agreed and called on the phone to make this request. Courtney was also present. She had just walked out of her courts in the public area and joined the conversation. Courtney seconded Sam's request with this new idea.

It was done! The tennis playing cards with my natural name John Riggio arrived. They were dispersed around to my fans. The effort Sam made helped another idea, and that was to correct the problems with the player name game I had gone through for a long time. I thanked him for the successful plea.

At some time playing at the Sutton East Tennis Center my tournament winning number started to add to a new discussion. The list of papers and ATP charts my sponsors possessed showed that the winning numbers I had totaled up to that time had made me an official "Tennis Legend". This was a great title for my pro tennis playing. Gloria told me this fact one day from the management office in the tennis center. This was just from numbers compiled through pieces of sports records that were unified in my contract trades. There were more and more match wins and tournament wins along with ATP records as a junior pro player and an adult pro player that weren't compiled.

Overall my playing with my sponsor Ms. Gloria Vanderbilt proved a great investment and profits for everyone. She had stated that her personal debts were over and she was out of bankruptcy. I was a proven sports business investment. The more money they made the more everyone believed in my playing greatness. She had compared me with baseball player Babe Ruth. This is because of my growing wins and clout in sports.

The ATP again put a hold on my contract and Gloria would have to hire a new Lawyer to keep my tennis playing going. Courtney's contract was also put on hold. Ms. Gloria Vanderbilt and Company were having a difficult time with the contract renewal. There was no real reason for the stop in my contract. My playing was great. I was an honest and sportsmanlike player.

Ms. Gloria Vanderbilt hired attorney Mr. Rudolph Gulliani. He was listed as the best Lawyer in NYC. Years later he would also become the Mayor of New York City. He was retained by Gloria to get a contract renewal for both of her players. I was told the Lawyers were working on my case.

I had to sue the National Tennis Center years before to curtail a playing stoppage. I did it myself and went to the courtroom in Queens, NYC against some of the players who were visible to me at the National Tennis Center. I won the case and that helped me continue playing for at least 5 years.

This case was really a reinstatement of the first case I had made. The lawyer Gloria hired was never fully aware of this situation. No one called me to testify at the lawyer office or in the courtroom. For Courtney, she was more intertwined by the Guiliani office and appeared in court at their request.

I was told after the court case that the Judge asked in the courtroom. "Where is John?". The lawyers didn't know what to say. The fact that this was a continuation of my original court case was uncovered. Since there was a miscommunication between the parties, the court case wasn't successful to renew the two contracts, the court litigation was abandoned.

The pressures from the sports litigation started to succumb to my contract with Ms. Gloria Vanderbilt and company. She decided to put my contract up for sale. The initial price was 25 Million Dollars. She offered the contract through sports business channels and we all waited for a reply.

With Vanderbilt's sponsorship, I became a powerhouse on the court, winning big tournaments and establishing myself among the best in the world. The story of my ascent in the world of professional tennis is not merely an account of victories and fame; it's also a chronicle of struggles, legal battles, contractual complexities, and the relentless pursuit of success. As my playing skills improved and the prize money increased, I faced a series of challenging hurdles that tested my resolve and resilience.

Chapter Seven
Moving Up and Outdoors

My contract started to face unexpected hurdles, as it was put on hold by the Association of Tennis Professionals (ATP) without clarification. My sponsors exhausted their help, and ran out of litigation attempts. Ms. Gloria Vanderbilt told me the names of some Lawyers to call and see if I can find help to close a deal on a new buyer of my tennis contract.

Finding a capable attorney became a priority. I reached out to the office of Mrs. Hillary Rodham Clinton, known not just for her political career as United States Secretary of State and the first lady to President Bill Clinton but also for her work as an Attorney, with high-profile contracts involving athletes and entertainers. To my relief, Hillary was interested in helping me with my contract situation. Through her adept handling and negotiations with Gloria Vanderbilt's group, she facilitated the sale of my contract.

To start the sale of my contract a marketing video was made. This included photographs and an introductory video of me playing on television. There were supporting documents of my playing stats. My pro tennis player trading card was an important part of the package.

The promotional package was sent to some interested investors in the sports business. There were some initial bids on the contract. The starting bid was 25 Million Dollars. As the agreement was negotiated the price didn't go down it went up. The price climbed to 30 Million Dollars—a substantial validation of my talent and marketability.

A successful negotiation was made and a lucrative deal of 30 Million Dollars was made. The frontman for the contract was Mr. Ross Perot. My new sponsor started to get involved with my tennis playing. To make this happen, my lawyer continued communicating with all sides involved. It was so big in money and diverse with so many lines of playing and advertising.

As the details of the final contract sale were worked out there was some time off from playing tennis. I was at home where I grew up and continued with all of the different things I had going with a College education and working a job to make some money to pay all of the bills I had. This wait time was seen as a vulnerable point where someone could ruin things for the contract sale and my pro tennis playing. To check on my well being some people were volunteering to see if I was ok. Since pro tennis at this level is not only big business but involves people in the US government. There were different people who came to check on me. One of them was the Senator, Mr. Joe Biden from Delaware who took a few minutes from his busy schedule and arrived at my home. Mr. Biden was later to attain the highest office of President of the United States of America. I talked to Mr. Biden right in front of my house, it was just an everyday discussion. He saw my age and neighborhood situation, then quickly decided to reference one of his sons to follow up with me. Just a few days later I had an appointment with Mr. Hunter Biden. Hunter arrived right on time, he had just made the long car trip direct from Delaware and arrived right in front of my house in Jericho, NY. He was about my same age and was able to relate to the whole picture of what was going on with my life. The start of my new tennis contract was of prime concern and I stayed in contact with him to assure a safe start to my tennis playing. I was finally called by my lawyer and given the start date and time of my tennis playing at the SUNY Old Westbury Tennis complex. Ahead of the start date, I called Hunter to update him on my tennis playing location, with the date and time. It was 7:30 am in the morning and I was on the tennis court's right on time to start hitting the ball with the other pros. As I looked over to the parking area Mr. Hunter Biden arrived at the courts to catch the opening day of the tennis playing. This was the start of the new contract with the Perot Group. Everything had worked out great and with the watching eyes of these people I didn't have problems before the matches started. It was overall a great success!

I was able to handle this move up in the contract. The new tennis court that was selected at the SUNY Old Westbury College Campus comprised 3 groups of tennis courts and an Athletic Building. I was playing on one reserved court. Next to my court there were metal bleachers and a walkway to the parking lot. The sponsors had security guards blocking the roads to the tennis complex. This was to make sure everyone was safe during the pro tennis playing.

To start playing with the Perot Group, there were 5 young pro players they were already sponsoring. This group helped me warm up my playing. Since there was a playing stoppage after Sutton East. It took a few matches to sharpen up my tennis playing ability. I was ready to play some pro matches. After I started to play some serious matches with the group of players, they had their coach come over to see for himself. He stood by the court side and watched the matches. Perot's coach was nice to point out anything about my playing that I could improve on. A pro player is always learning and improving. As the matches went on, he watched me play one of his players after another. After I won one match, the coach asked me "Who won the match?" I answered "I did." He repeatedly pointed his finger to himself and replied "NO! I DID!!!". He thought he had taught all of his players how to win the tennis matches.

When I started playing with this new sponsor the name John Vanderbilt was gone and a new tennis player name was getting formulated. The new tennis manager from Perot was there and he gave me a choice of using the name John Vice or Carlos Scipio. I told him I like the name John Vice. This name was simple and easy to pronounce. The manager made a mental note of it, but a few days later he told me I have to use Carlos Scipio. I was to later find out the reason why. The name was selected by a marketing company, who did research with tennis spectators around the world. This research made everyone believe the name Carlos Scipio could get advertised to different parts of the world. I was told that my player name did get marketed around the world and my tennis player name was successful.

Perot was really making a big investment into my contract and wanted to start expanding my sports advertising. Since my new name Carlos Scipio was finalized, there was the next desire to have a spokesman. The spokesman would go on radio or television to answer questions. This would bring my image to the world of sports spectators around the world. The first spokesman came to my tennis court. He told me about himself and we played some tennis. He didn't work out and was replaced with a new spokesman. The next spokesman also met at my court. He introduced himself and we played some tennis. This spokesman was eager to start work and stayed on the job.

The next part of my contract was to have a stand-in. The stand-in met me at my court. He also introduced himself and we played some tennis. The stand-in was different from the spokesman. He was sized to look just like me and was marked with a tattoo on his arm. The next thing he needed to learn was how to act like me. I showed him some gestures I usually do. After that he needed to learn how to play tennis like me. I showed him some playing style so he would play similar to me on the court. He told me he might travel places and stand-in on the tennis court, hit the ball and more. This was a marketing idea to travel and have my playing seen in different areas of the world. I was told later this idea worked with great success.

Navigating these new relationships grew complicated, especially when facing the potential overshadowed by my stand-in who attempted to mimic my persona during events. Although these decisions came from a place of overwhelming business acumen, the risk of diluting my identity and authenticity added layers of concern to my burgeoning career.

The next marketing need was to have a fancy car. The manager of the Perot sponsors knew the McLaren Car group. I talked to the car leaser and he was so enthralled by my pro tennis playing arrangements that agreed to have a new F1 at the courtside. The car was so fast it required a special training class to drive.

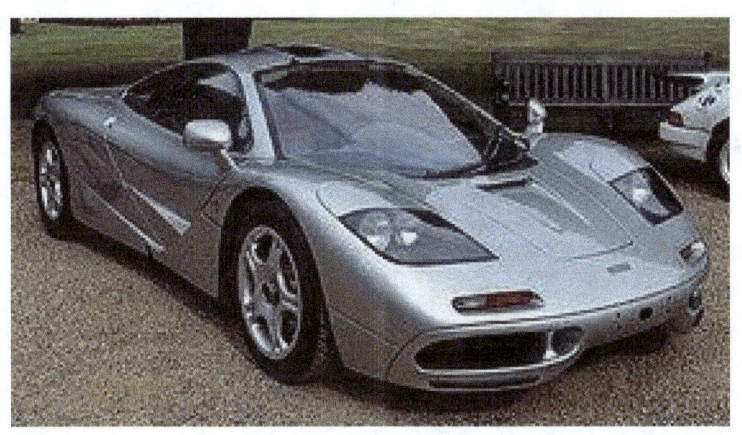

Photo: 1990 McLaren F1 car.

I was playing tennis at the courts starting at 7:30 am and ending at 7:30 pm. There were a lot of matches to play. As I played there Mr. Ross Perot arrived by helicopter. He landed right on top of the closest hill next to the tennis complex. I saw him and he talked to me from a distance. He waved over to me and I waved back. From a distance he shouted over to me and said a number of things. He welcomed me as the star tennis player he was sponsoring and thought things were going great. They were going great. Perot championed my tennis playing and knew I was a great investment. He also knew about my tennis stadium they started building in the north part of Manhattan, NYC, but said he didn't want to finish building the stadium because of a previous stadium venture he was involved with in the State of Texas. He also said tennis wasn't a stadium sport. After Mr. Perot finished visiting the SUNY Old Westbury tennis complex, he got back into his helicopter and flew away.

These new experiences required me to talk to my lawyer on a regular basis. The next part of my contract was having a nice girlfriend present. At courtside there were some other females with a contract the same size. I used to talk to them and exchange personal contact information.

I told my lawyer the story about how Dahlia is my girlfriend and she liked watching my tennis matches. She was allowed to come to my court a few times. She was very happy to see my pro playing continue to move up. I used to meet Dahlia at her house after the matches. This was at 9 pm at night and I used to wake up early so I was back on the tennis courts by 7:30 am the next day.

Dahlia couldn't get enough of watching my tennis playing at Old Westbury. Her desire to attend my tennis matches was great. On one occasion she was jumping up and down so happy with the live video panning over and recording her.

From a check-in with my lawyer, I was told the Perot Group already marketed my contract. They were successful in finding a new sports investor. The new investor was Mitsubishi Japan. I was told some players were going to meet me at Old Westbury and play some tournaments.

The team from Japan arrived and the playing was very good. They had a coach that monitored the group. I was playing great as usual. I won every match. The coach the Japan team had wasn't taking it well and threatened to start cheating. This coach was later reprimanded for his behavior.

There was one tournament, the Nippon Open. They really put a lot of effort into this. There was court signage, ball boys and a judge stand. I played through this very confidently. The last few matches were internationally televised. I won the final match and the tournament.

The tournament was from far away and the tournament was imported from far away. The television was going direct to Japan. I was exhilaratingly happy when my neighbor Mr. Hy Ozer emerged from his front door and congratulated me on winning the Nippon Open.

With the tennis team from Japan was the team from South Korea, Indonesia, Taiwan, Guam, and the

Philippines. In addition to these teams, the best male tennis player from mainland China was present and playing in the tournaments. Each team traveled by airplane to New York City. They were then brought by coach bus to my court in Old Westbury. I could see groups of them unloading and walking to the waiting area. The Indonesian team arrived with two coach buses.

The tennis teams were happy to play me. They didn't get angry if I won a match. I won all of the tennis matches. This probably made their trip worth their while, knowing they traveled a long distance to play the number 1 player. After all of my matches were finished, I offered to teach them tennis as the tournaments ended. I explained this idea is a standard in the USA and was already teaching students for the National Tennis Center. They agreed and I started to teach some of their players.

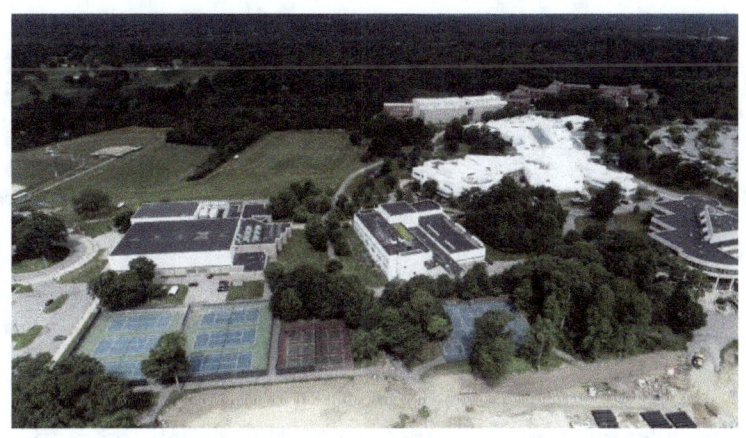

Photo: SUNY Old Westbury tennis complex.

The Pacific tennis teams started to leave the courts and were on their way back home. I noticed that all of the teams from the Pacific came to meet me but didn't play with the National Tennis Center. The players from the National Tennis Center would have to travel to Japan on their own to play tournaments.

The next round of tennis tournaments for me was the players from the National Tennis Center. The Perot sponsor was hoping for good results. I started to play some tournaments with an assortment of matches televised. All of these matches were on my own courts at Old Westbury. I started to win the matches as usual. With the match wins came the tournament wins and the big money for my sponsors.

Throughout my development in tennis, the landscape has remained one of contrasts. On the one hand, a commitment to ethical play propelled me forward, while on the other, a cast of characters highlighted the lengths some would go to win unjustly.

During this set of tournaments, I had often communicated with my lawyer. Comparing my game-playing record on the court didn't match the written record with the ATP. One of the tournaments was won by a player that had corrupt sponsors. He was also assisting in the crime of grand larceny. He and his sponsors fooled the ATP to give them the trophy and the prize money. After my account of the match score and the meticulous review of the videotape proved I won the matches and the tournament. The trophy sent to the fraudulent player was returned to my sponsor Perot. The prize money was also returned and sent to my sponsors. The fraudulent opponent and his organization was charged with grand larceny. I was later told they were convicted.

The weather in the Northeast of the United States started to get colder and the daylight ended earlier in the fall season. My tennis playing was planned to get relocated from the SUNY Old Westbury courts to the new indoor tennis center in Glenwood Landing, NY. This was a twenty-minute drive from the Old Westbury courts. I drove over and visited the indoor tennis facility a few times. The building was getting renovated to start my winter playing. I would continue to have my own court.

I played all of the ATP Players that are usually seen at the US Open. They couldn't beat me. I won all of the tournaments against them. As the Japan team watched me play they all started to warm up to the fact that the players from the National Tennis Center couldn't win against me either. The team from Japan was relieved. As they learned that Mitsubishi Japan bought my contract they were starting to root for me.

One important match that was televised was against one of the top players coming out of the green building at the National Tennis Center. This is the group of players people usually see when watching the US Open in Queens, NY. The team from Japan and the Mitsubishi sponsors were present to watch the match. It was part of an ATP tournament that I would later win. As I played the match with great confidence my new sponsors were getting excited. I had excellent serves, my net play was perfect. I was hitting the ball to the left of my opponent then to the right of my opponent. With my Babolat pro stock tennis racket I was hitting the ball very well. My opponent tried to make an effort to stop my advance in the match. In his push to get the ball and hit it back over the net, he fell on the court's hard surface. I really made the crowd stand in awe! From my precision playing, I clearly took control of the game and won big. I could see the Japan sponsors and teammates jumping up and down in joy, as I played great tennis. They already started to win big too, as new sponsors for my pro tennis playing.

I checked with my lawyer Ms. Hillary Clinton. She started to tell me the most amazing thing about my career. Mitsubishi Japan has decided to buy my contract for 100 Million US dollars. This is the biggest contract in tennis history. My contract surpassed the previous number one contract holder Mr. Guillermo Vilas. He had a 80 Million Dollar contract. Guillermo, who is 16 years older than me, was present to play me in some tournament matches at the Old Westbury courts.

As a requirement of the US Contract Law both my player name and the 100 Million Dollar contract amount were listed in the *Newsday* paper's sports section in NYC and surrounding suburbs. It was also listed in a Los

Angeles, CA newspaper. For additional US Law reasons, my name was listed as Ron Devlin in NYC. In L.A. it was said to have a listing of Carlos Scipio. The only other sports players above me on that list were Jose Conseco in Baseball, Michael Jordan in Basketball and Magic Johnson in Basketball. My contract amount was listed per year but the other contracts were listed per a 3 year term. We didn't complain about the contract listing parameters. My top contract in Tennis was the most important.

The summit of my contracts saw my worth escalate to astounding figures, with contracts soaring to a whopping 100 Million Dollars. All the while, my identity remained under scrutiny, dictated by people who had little to do with my personal integrity.

At these heights, my relationship with Hillary Clinton became pivotal. Not only did she navigate the complexities of sports contracts, but she also provided legal support during turbulent moments. However, the necessity of having a proper agent emerged as another pivotal struggle. I sought out agents adept at navigating entertainment deals. Yet, my preliminary inquiries led to frustrations, as many agents were elusive or hesitant to take on a tennis player whose star was still rising.

I made some efforts at this time to have a better agent to collect my sports earnings. Even having Dahlia's father as my agent was forwarded as a solution. The funds by default would go to my parents unless I could establish more independent management of my career.

Simultaneously, a publicist became necessary to bolster my image and ensure that I was featured in the right circles. With previous attempts yielding mixed results, I resolved to secure a top-notch publicist, a task that proved to be more challenging than I anticipated. Establishing the right publicity channels was essential if I aspired to elevate my career akin to other athletes whose narratives filled tabloids and sports news.

Faced with the enormity of the struggles, I learned that a successful contract can attract the interest of both a spokesman and a stand-in, individuals devoted to preserving my public persona. While initially accommodating, The culmination of these factors reached a critical point when my contract was valued at an unprecedented 100 Million Dollars.

All the while, I knew my journey was far from simple; it became a constant balancing act. The myriad intricacies of sponsorships, contracts, publicity amidst personal relationships reflected how the world of professional tennis was a complicated tapestry full of vibrant colors, with shadows lurking just beneath the surface. As I learned more about the business side of my sport, it became clear that my professional ambitions would require not just skillful playing but also shrewd navigation of the complexities that came with fame and fortune.

Chapter Eight
An International View

It is the end of winter and my new sponsor from Japan, Mitsubishi Sports, called me on the telephone. They greeted me with the name Mr. Carlos Scipio. My natural name was put aside with these telephone conversations. My new sponsors were different from the previous sponsors I had worked with. This new player name assigned to me was very stringently used. Carlos Scipio became my real name for now. They asked me to play along with this idea. They had primarily two sports administrators that I talked to. The first administrator was the so-called Coach of the team from Japan. Unfortunately, this Coach wasn't compatible. This was the same Coach that was the Chair Umpire during the tennis matches in Old Westbury. He would sit in a wooden stand during the matches. On the raised chair he looked at me and made a statement that if his players couldn't win against me, then he would start to cheat.

My tournament wins against the players from the National Tennis Center had overridden their anger and made them put aside their hurt feelings.

As I communicated with the first Coach he didn't have any sponsor knowhow. The Coach also had a temperamental personality and instead of just arranging the tennis matches, he started yelling on the phone. He was a unique personality in tennis up to now. He wasn't a former pro tennis player and was instead college educated in the sports industry.

In a desperate effort, we tried to coordinate a trip to Japan. This involved me driving to Laguardia Airport, located in Queens, NYC and walking into Japan Air terminal. The Coach's declaration that I would receive an airplane ticket to travel to Japan was wrong. From many drives back and forth to Japan Air I started to keep my suitcase in my car. I was changing my clothes out of my suitcase during each weekday. I did this so I could drive to the airport with a short notice, park my car and board the airplane. I finally went there with $1,000 cash and bought a one way airline ticket. The only problem was I needed a Visa to travel to Japan back then. The ticket desk at Japan Air called their travel agent but a Visa wasn't available.

There was confusion over a professional sports Visa or a simple travel Visa. The Japan Air office didn't issue either. Japan Air talked to the Coach in Japan on the telephone. He didn't know what to do. This was a first for him. The ticket desk refunded my money for the air fare.

I have traveled before and obviously, this kind of direct ticket and travel wasn't working. The Coach from the Japanese sponsors didn't have the know-how. I noticed the money wasn't there either.

I had many call backs with my lawyer, Ms. Hillary Clinton. Since the Coach from the Japanese sponsors couldn't start my playing in the USA or Japan there was a big problem brewing. My lawyer took action with the International Sports Court. This Court is part of the United Nations. They started an investigation into Mitsubishi Japan's conduct with my pro tennis playing contract. They determined that Mitsubishi, Japan was in violation of a few things. One serious violation was the Coach from Japan had me play too many matches for too many hours per day. Since he was in a rush to play all of the matches in a short time at Old Westbury, NY, he had me start playing at 7:30 am and end playing at 7:30 pm. This was considered an abuse of a professional Athlete. The usual rule was a pro player can play 3 days a week for 5 hours each day maximum. They also determined Mitsubishi had about six months to get my pro tennis playing on the courts. Since they couldn't come through with arranging any ATP tennis matches, they were again in violation. They were also in violation of never sending my representatives the minimum pro tennis salary I should earn for the year.

From this discovery of violations including the timed out playing, the Mitsubishi Japan sponsors were fined 400 Million US dollars Plus fees by the International Court. Mitsubishi paid the full penalty to the USA. It was the largest settlement for sports contracts in the world. This was talked about in political news shows on national television stations in the USA. The violations of my pro tennis playing additionally resulted in a suspension of 7 years for Japan's international sports investing.

Japan's representatives also helped with the judgement and arrested the Coach that didn't have the knowhow and forced the long hours of playing. The Coach was sentenced to many months in prison. Since Japan paid the fine and arrested the Coach they were in full compliance. This allowed an agreement with the International Court to keep my pro tennis contract open indefinitely.

I then started to talk to Mitsubishi Japan's next tennis Coach and sports Administrator, Mr. Shigeyuki Nishio. He did superb work compared to his predecessor. Mr. Nishio wasn't just a tennis Administrator but was also a pro tennis player for many years, and is well known throughout Japan. Shigeyuki was there to continue a line of communication with Mitsubishi, this kept the phone conversations with Japan going. I started to broaden my understanding of tennis from around the world. Japan agreed that playing in a stadium wasn't the centerpoint of their game, they didn't consider tennis a stadium sport. We did discuss the sports car affixation and they have the fancy cars around the pro sport players. The whole thing with players having side jobs was also a standard in Japan, many players even take to working as an Architectural draftsman. The excitement of pro tennis kept them involved in the game.

By staying in contact with my sponsors in Japan, I was able to find out the previous Coach from Mitsubishi decided to commit suicide before he could serve his prison sentence.

The next plan was to play local matches. From my input I had my sponsors in Japan contact some local tennis administrative coach in the USA. I had called around to different tennis people and gained some hints at Japan playing in the USA. One was for Mitsubishi Sports to file business papers in the USA to gain a local office with employees. This local establishment would in theory arrange legal pro ATP matches for my tennis playing.

There were additional efforts to find sports knowhow to get my pro matches going. I suggested an investor in Japan who is involved in the sports business. My Japanese sponsors did know someone and they gave me his phone number. I took my chances and called the businessman. My efforts were a success. After my call was forwarded from the secretary I discussed my pro tennis playing for Mitsubishi. My phone calls to this businessman wasn't a waste of time. He was interested as an investor but didn't run the tennis matches. Since I showed a desire to have Japan make money on my contract, he became very impressed with my personality. He gave me some insights on improving my life, I was ready for anything and I tried his suggestions out. The CEO asked that I give him a phone call when I start playing tennis matches again.

With the local matches still in the works, my Japan sponsors planned an extended visit to Japan for me. I would stay in the Olympic apartments they have available for up to four years. They promised to cover the rent and basic needs. The only catch was I needed to bring my girlfriend Dahlia. I told them about Dahlia and this was their one condition on this new venture to Japan.

I asked my girlfriend Dahlia and she said "yes". The only problem was she had to receive permission from her father to make the journey to Japan. Her father could even travel with us for a shorter stay. I met Dahlia at her house, her father was present and told me "no". He said he was born in Shanghai, China and doesn't like Japanese people. With outrage he spoke up and said he wants a company like Samsung and not Mitsubishi to own my tennis contract. With these serious problems, my new trip to Japan was put on hold.

I had checked back with my Lawyer and was given an update. My spokesman was no longer in the tennis contract. My stand-in was also removed from my contract. The stand-in started to take on a life of his own and changed his last name. His first name remained the same as Carlos and he is still playing pro tennis somewhere.

One player who was born in the Philippines but usually played in Japan because he was an up-and-coming pro really took to my training at Old Westbury. He was eager to learn to play better tennis and saw that my offer to teach tennis was of great value. He was an excellent student and really started to improve at a pro level of tennis playing. I was told after he returned back to Japan he continued to play better. He won one pro tournament against some of the best tennis players. This victory was attributed to my teaching him tennis at Old Westbury. His better percentage of winning started to make waves in pro tennis. His improved playing was again proof of my great tennis playing, and my ability to teach pro players how to win matches.

Months went by and I decided to talk to one of my pro sports and entertainment friends, Mimi. The idea of traveling to Hawaii came about. From some input with my friend on Hawaii, the idea of going there could work. I then called Mr. Shigeyuki Nishio and started to discuss this idea with him. He was very happy with the travel idea and told me they have some players from Japan in Hawaii. I was finally making progress getting the pro tennis playing going and the travel dates were set.

Dahlia was included in this new travel plan. I asked her to come along and she said "yes". I had the whole trip planned with my local travel agent. Dahlia filled out the travel agent forms and signed at the bottom. She was eager to make the trip to Hawaii. I paid the money for our reservations and had our tickets ready to go. Unfortunately, Dahlia's father stopped the trip again. This time it was worse. He threatened to refrain from giving Dahlia her money from the conservatory. Dahlia's father claimed to have set up a savings account called a conservatory. This was a sort of inheritance where she could gain control of funds at some time in the future. He was also saying he doesn't trust the Japanese and thought they were just lying to me.

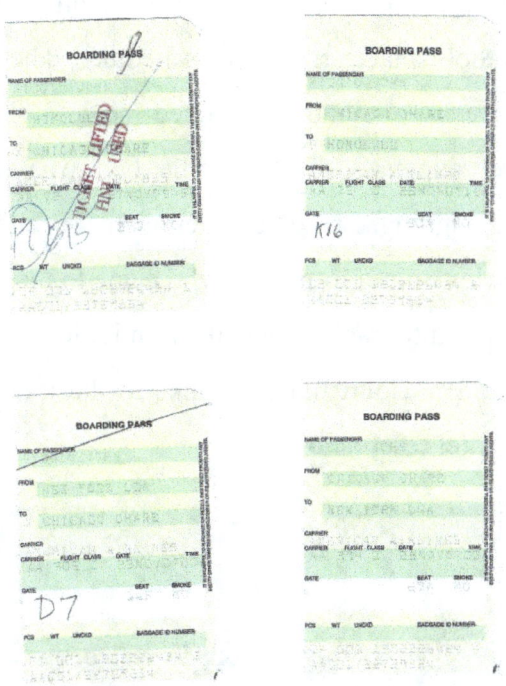

Photo: Airline boarding passes to Hawaii 1995.

I wouldn't let Dahlia stop my trip! Since there was no requirement for Dahlia to attend with me, I traveled to Hawaii on my own and on the same dates as planned. I arrived in Honolulu, HI on November 23, 1995, and stayed at a very nice high-rise hotel called the Maile Sky Court. The next day, I made new friends at the hotel. I toured around the island of Honolulu and went to the beach.

The date and time to meet my Japanese sponsors in Hawaii took place right on schedule. The Mitsubishi contact greeted me and reimbursed me in cash dollars for the travel expenses. The idea he had was to make an autograph signing. I received a tennis racket and signed my name Carlos Scipio to people who came to the event. I was signing my autographs right in the middle of the lobby of the Maile Sky Court hotel. Thanks to the travel agent for the nice hotel reservation.

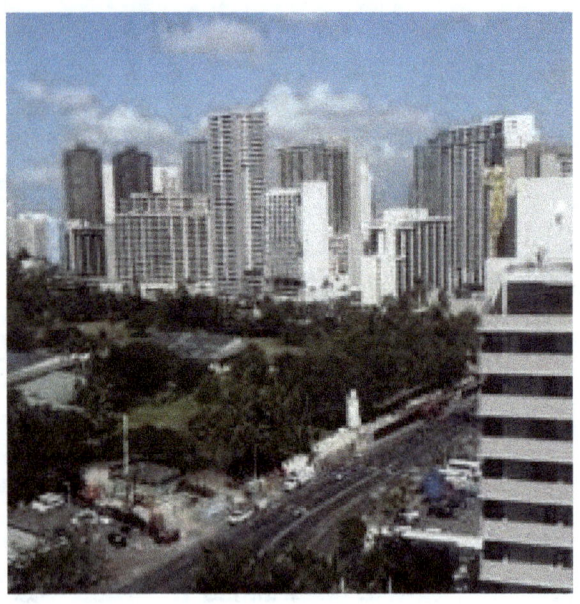

Photo: Maile Sky Court Hotel in Honolulu, Hawaii.

The sponsor then introduced me to music entertainer Ms. Gwen Stefani. She had her group of female singers with her called the Harajuku Girls. I was invited to attend her concert in Honolulu, HI that same night. Professional photographers took some photos in the lobby.

The sponsor introduced me to one of the tennis players associated with Mitsubishi. We talked about playing tennis in Hawaii. He told me the location of some tennis courts they had available.

Everything was ok to return and play some matches in Hawaii. The trip was a great success for meeting my sponsors. I also signed autographs the next morning at the same hotel lobby where I was staying. The tennis event was finished for this trip. The minivan arrived and drove me to the Airport. I returned home with no problems.

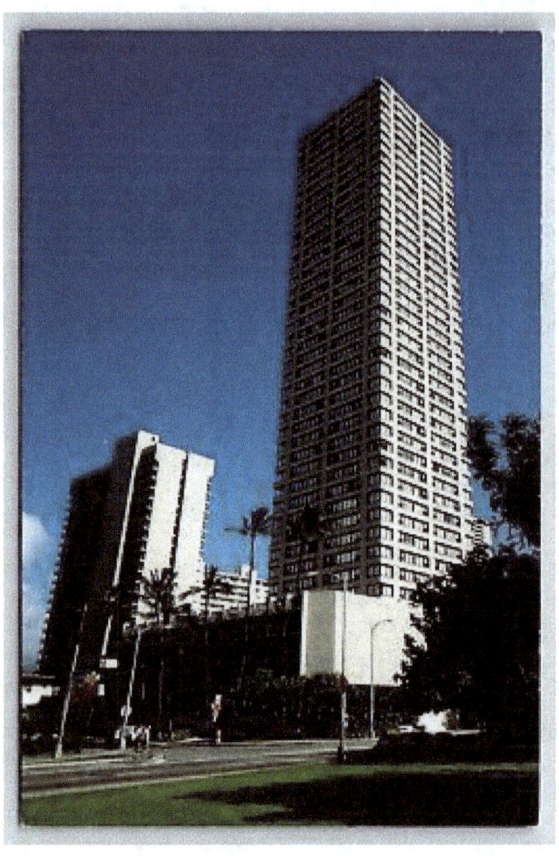

Photo: Maile Sky Court Hotel in Honolulu, Hawaii.

After the new year in 1996, I talked to Dahlia in the Broadway Mall where she worked. I told her my trip was a great success and showed her proof of the events at the hotel. Some of her friends were so ecstatic about the introduction with Ms. Gwyn Stephanie. They also really started to believe in my tennis greatness. I offered Dahlia to travel with me for a second trip to Hawaii. Instead of acting so happy she became enraged at her father who had stopped the previous two trips to meet the Japanese sponsors. She felt let down by her father and was just played a fool.

Dahlia ran as fast as she could out of the Mall to confront her father. This was the last time I saw my girlfriend Dahlia. I had first met her in Kindergarten and then held a long relationship with her ever since I signed the pro tennis contract with Mr. Anthony Cambria.

I followed up by visiting Dahlia's house but no one was living there anymore. As I rang the front door bell, the nice old lady from next door walked over to me. She was a familiar face, Me and Dahlia used to talk to her in front of Dahlia's house a number of times over the years. The neighbor liked us together as a couple and thought we should get married. She didn't like the other boys Dahlia knew. The lady next door told me her recollection of what happened.

It seems the confrontation between Dahlia and her father resulted in her death. From knowing Dahlia's home problems there were security cameras all over her house. A few weeks later I met Dahlia's best friend in the Mall and she told me there was a funeral and Dahlia's casket was closed. I wasn't invited to the funeral. The death of Dahlia was hard on me and everyone she knew.

More than a year later, some of Dahlia's friends in the Mall told me her father was found dead in Florida. He was already getting involved with bad things and it ended in his demise.

Dahlia always helped my career. Our unofficial marriage was based on keeping tennis and entertainment at the forefront. We loved each other and keeping our adventure going was paramount. She was also my best spectator. She had the best percentage of seeing me win 100 percent of the matches she sat in on. In the very first match, she watched me play. I saw her from a distance to the school tennis courts. She had ridden her bicycle there on her own and waved over. This wasn't an easy match and I made a comeback effort to win.

My tennis playing was never based on Dahlia. Learning tennis started when I was very young with my family. My playing abilities were all there and I was still eager to keep playing pro tennis, even with these horrible problems around me. Starting on my own again, I thought in my mind really hard! I tried to figure out how my pro tennis playing could continue using the knowledge I already had. I called the head office of Mitsubishi and described the situation in the USA with pro tennis playing. The female employee really took my advice and was learning very quickly from my instructions on how new sponsors to my contract can make my pro tennis revive. She was able to search for an investor and found Mr. Bernie Tapie, a businessman who owned Adidas Sporting Goods. The office worker told me she had an interested investor but couldn't make the deal by herself. To solve this problem I requested Mitsubishi call my lawyer Ms. Hillary Clinton. They agreed with this idea and the employee was invigorated about the reference.

I followed up with my lawyer Ms. Hillary Clinton and was able to find out the details of Adidas's interest in my contract. I also found out that Reebok Sporting Goods, in Britain, was also investing in my contract. I later checked with the Mitsubishi office and found out my contract was increased to 120 Million US Dollars. Reebok was made the main contact in the new investment. I was told to wait for the new representative from Reebok to call me directly on the telephone.

It was just a short wait and I answered the phone call from the apartment I was living in. The Reebok representative and myself talked on the telephone about my new sponsorship. He was calling from Britain and wasn't fully knowledgeable about tennis playing in the USA. To help start the playing, I gave him the phone numbers to call the National Tennis Center.

He didn't wait on the tennis playing. I received a time date and location to play a pro match. From my apartment, I drove to the tennis court, and another pro player showed up. We warmed up by hitting the ball. To my disappointment, my opponent told me he was directed to only come out to hit the ball. He wasn't allowed to play a full match. He then had to leave and drove away. The next pro-matches Reebok setup were very similar. Finally in one of these tennis meetings, I was told by my opponent that it was my Sponsor who didn't set up the match correctly. He had previously asked what the story was with the playing arrangements before he arrived that afternoon. This new statement made a big difference. I called back to Reebok and informed him of the problem.

The other pro players were also commenting that arranging a pro tennis match on such a simple tennis court wasn't good for this level of playing. They wanted a tennis center to play in. I understood what they were saying. The locations that were selected just had a few open tennis courts with no building, lockers, bathroom or anything around. There were just open fields visible. I didn't have a say in the new locations to meet at.

Reebok couldn't solve the problems with the National Tennis Center. I quickly tried contacting some previous sponsors. Upon calling Ms. Gloria Vanderbilt I told her that my contract price had reached 120 Million Dollars and my lead sponsors were Reebok and Adidas. I also explained my predicament with my match playing getting stalled out. Ms. Vanderbilt was very impressed with my contract and sponsors. The only problem was she sold my contract years ago and wasn't allowed to buy it back. Gloria thought about some available investors and gave me Ms. Leona Helmsley' phone number as a reference. There was a chance she would agree to a new sports investment.

Chapter Nine
My Last Big Tournament Run

Miss Leona Helmsley, was an influential figure in New York City. She was also the wife of Harry Helmsley, a wealthy hotel businessman. This is the family I was referenced to by Ms. Gloria Vanderbilt. I wrote down the phone number and called Ms. Helmsley's office. The deskman answered and I simply explained that I am a professional tennis player and available for a new sponsorship.

The message was forwarded and I started to talk with Ms. Leona Hemlsley directly. She was very interested in sponsoring me. The only provision she had was my age, 28 years old, and the price of my contract, 120 Million Dollars. She needed more information about my pro tennis playing and wanted some recommendations for the sponsorship. This direct phone call was high stakes for me, but I knew I could come through to win big.

The next step was to call Ms. Gloria Vanderbilt back to gain some supporting recommendations and reply to Ms.

Helmsley. Gloria immediately communicated with Leona and gave me a recommendation for my pro tennis playing. Gloria also devised a plan to show proof of my tennis greatness. The plan was to have me play some demonstration matches for Ms. Helmsley at the Sutton East Tennis Center in Manhattan, NYC.

I hadn't played at Sutton East in 4 years. It was good to return to a safe large tennis center in the middle of Manhattan, NYC. As I walked into the tennis center I remembered all of the great times I had. I was full of confidence and met Gloria and Ms. Leona Helmsley. Ms. Helmsley's husband Harry was there too. I was greeted by my new sponsors and we talked about the tennis matches ahead.

I was 28 years old but still thin and in great shape. My last physical exam was excellent. I only had 6 percent body fat. My exercise schedule was the usual jogging and bicycle riding. I did work out with some weights, but not too much.

I walked onto my old tennis court and looked around, noticing the bright lights of the bubble. I reacquainted myself with playing on the court. As I waited there my opponent finally arrived. He was sent by the National Tennis Center and it was an ATP match. We started to play the match. I was playing excellently and my shots were still tight. My opponent didn't play as well and started to cheat. He called my passing shots out repeatedly. I had to stop the match and complain. As he repeatedly committed the same cheating, I stopped the match and protested my opponent's behavior to Ms. Vanderbilt. My opponent was also using his racket in a strange way. Leaning back to hit the ball. It was obviously a cheat racket. This is an illegally made tennis racket strung to 73 lbs.

My sponsor stopped the match and asked my opponent to leave the court. My opponent's tennis racket was inspected and the information about the racket was written down. Some phone calls were made. My opponent was asked to leave the Sutton East Tennis Center.

As I exited the tennis center I talked to Leona and Gloria. They asked me about Dahlia and hoped we were still together. I had to tell them the unfortunate news that Dahlia passed away because of her father. They were both in shock about this horrible news.

The next matches were scheduled. At the Sutton East Tennis Center, Mrs. Leona Helmsley watched me play more tennis matches. I was happy to find out that Ms.

Helmsley decided to invest in my contract. She contacted her lawyers and they started to negotiate a buy.

At this time I called Reebok in Britain and informed the tennis administrator about Ms. Leona Helmsley's wish to invest in my pro tennis contract. He was happy and said the Reebok company's lawyers would talk with the new investors.

I continued to play pro matches at the Sutton East Tennis Center again. I was winning big. Leona talked to me and told me her lawyers and the lawyers from Reebok couldn't come to an agreement. She asked me to call my lawyer to help with the contract investment.

I gave my lawyer Mrs. Hillary Rodham Clinton a phone call. She was able to come through again with some agreement proposals. The first proposal was a 60 Million Dollar investment to the 120 Million Dollar contract. This will make the new contract 180 Million Dollars. That first agreement didn't get approved because the lead sponsor Reebok would only give Ms. Helmsley a small percentage of the winnings.

The next proposal was a lease agreement. Where Ms. Leona Helmsley would pay a certain amount of money per month. This worked better since a larger percentage of the winnings would go to the Helmsley's. The agreement was finalized by my lawyer and my playing continued.

Ms. Gloria Vanderbilt noticed that my lawyer Ms. Hillary Clinton always came through with an agreement. No sponsor deal had fallen through since I knew Ms. Clinton. Gloria was very impressed and gave high praise to my lawyer equating her to how I always come through to win pro tennis matches and tournaments for my sponsors. All of this sports business was building up into a lot of money for everyone.

To start off playing with the new agreement the name Carlos Scipio was put aside and a new player name was made. The name "John Strong" was decided by Ms. Helmsley. The reason is I am seen as acting really strong. The usual player routine of advertisements and autograph signings weren't there yet. The fancy car wasn't so important at this time either.

My tennis playing was so excellent that I started to win big ATP tournaments. When I talked to Leona at the Sutton East Tennis Center she was so happy. She told me about some dollar amounts with the winnings after I won each tournament. This gave me an indication of my move up.

Ms. Helmsley wanted to give me a great experience playing pro tennis at Sutton East Tennis Center. Part of that was helping my personal life at the pro level. She was nice enough to match me with a potential girlfriend and wife. I talked to a few candidates to fit that goal. They were all very nice ladies. I was also hoping to meet an eligible female to bond with. Only some girlfriends could relate to pro tennis and entertainment. The idea of meeting a nice female for marriage was also backed by an idea of working in the Hotel industry and gaining an excellent income. She knew I was making money as an Architect, but the Hotel business was said to carry a higher pay and an administrative position.

I called back to my original Japan sponsor, Mr. Shigeyuki Nishio, and told him the good news. I also called the Japanese Businessman and informed them of my playing run in the USA. Since Mitsubishi was still in the contract they could make more money by investing in my games. They were happy about the change in my fortune. Just because of the faulty head coach in Japan, I tried my best to have the contract make a lot of money. From the new winnings they should have covered their initial investment and have a large profit.

The winnings of the playing started to become so large that the Reebok company found out and had to contact my Lawyer. I found out later the lease deal was quickly changed to a big investment of 20 Million Dollars by Ms. Leona Helmsley. The percentage of the profit stayed the same. This kept the pro playing going strong.

I checked in with my lawyer Ms. Hillary Clinton. I was updated about my total contract price. It was now 140 Million Dollars Plus. This is because the lease payments plus the 20 Million Dollars boosted the total up. I was still the highest contract and the number #1 player.

I was winning against players 10 years younger than me. They admitted I didn't play old and was still the top pro player. In one tournament final I played Mr. Jonas Svensson from years ago at the Fischer Open. I can still play great and was able to win the match and the tournament again.

In January of 1997, I was told that Mr. Harry Helmsey died at the age of 87 years old. This caused a big problem with my playing. My playing could stop because Ms. Helmsley was mourning the death of her husband and was unavailable to manage my matches at Sutton East Tennis Center.

To solve the problem in the immediate time frame. The ATP allowed each member of the tennis sponsors to watch a certain number of tournaments. This kept my playing going and I was able to win more matches and more tournaments.

The building manager helped with some matches, the administrative coach helped with some tournaments, and others helped with the matches.

I walked into the Sutton East Tennis Center in the morning and Ms. Leona Helmsley was back in the management office. She told me Mr. Harry Hemlsley's "Will" was settled and she is no longer in control of my Pro Tennis Contract. This decision was disappointing for me and Ms. Hemsley. We were winning big and I was forging a new future at a pro level. The contract was placed in control of Mr. Helmsley descendants. I was told I had to wait for the young Mr. Helmsley to decide what they wanted to do.

I still played for a short time. The first message I received was: The beneficiaries don't want to do anything with the contract. This caused a big uproar at the Sutton East Tennis Center and the Helmsley's beneficiaries reconsidered. In a change of heart, they decided to continue the contract. I was to start playing for the young Mr. Helmsley.

The playing wasn't as continuous as before. I met the young Mr. Helmsley and he told me his ideas on my playing contract. He was going to put my contract on sale for 190 Million Dollars. A short time later he told me that he might have an investor. I would have to stop playing and wait for a phone call.

The phone call did happen in just a short time. The new investor was Mr. Kellogg from the Kellogg Company. A family that founded the food manufacturer of breakfast cereal. I returned to Sutton East Tennis Center and the same uncertainty was there. He realized I was 31 years old and my contract was 140 Million Dollars. The young Mr. Helmsley stopped in to help Mr. Kellogg. This worked until the name of the investor was switched over to Mr. Kellogg.

Another phone call to my lawyer Ms. Hillary Clinton gave me the new numbers. My contract was now 150 Million Dollars Plus. Mr. Kellogg had invested 10 Million Dollars to increase my contract price. Everyone was still in on the percentage of winnings. This included Mitsubishi Japan.

I started to play ATP pro tournaments with Mr. Kellogg. The matches were at Sutton East Tennis Center. I had to play some warmup matches to sharpen my game. Mr. Kellogg wasn't that experienced as a tennis sponsor. The young Mr. Helmsley helped him to start the tournament playing but that was just a start. I suggested he hire an administrative coach to help with the pro playing. He did hire one coach. The only thing is this coach was used to helping tennis players at the end of their career. There was no change in how we played the tournaments. The one admission of truth the Coach made was that from the written books I was 250 ranking levels higher than the US Open pro tennis players. I was still the top player.

Mr. Kellogg then decided to summon the knowledge of Mr. Tony Scolnick to help with the tennis pro playing. He already was my administrative coach with Ms. Vanderbilt and was able to maximize my playing. His excellent work made my tennis playing stable for a while. As the tennis playing became a regular occurrence at the Sutton East Tennis Center, Mr. Kellogg asked me about the tennis playing and the tennis center environment. I told him from previous experience, there were all kinds of things he could add on; like a return of the fan club, advertisements in local newspapers, autograph signing events, fancy cars on display, live television cameras, ATP awards, etc. Also without the grandstand at the Sutton East Tennis Center, all of the spectators couldn't join in the fun for some of the big matches.

Mr. Kellogg did listen to my advice for turning the place back on. He parked a nice sports car in front of the tennis center. He also started to add some more things on the list I had just blurted out.

It seems every time I won a Pro Tournament my sponsors were receiving threats against them. He took measures to hire security guards, etc. A sponsor's job is very difficult and can be dangerous. I had excellent sponsors that could stop cheating and other distractions and threats. Mr. Kellogg was no different than my previous sponsors. He was younger than my other sponsors and was learning as the matches continued on. From all the pressures and dangers in sports business he was becoming disenfranchised with investing in sports and thought he was going to stop doing this kind of business. Mr. Kellogg told me he was going on vacation at the end of 1997 and was going to refresh his mind and make a decision on the sport business. I was to continue playing some more tennis starting in January of 1998.

Over the holiday season I didn't tell anyone I was even playing any tennis. The phone call came and I returned back to the Sutton East Tennis Center to play tennis in January of 1998 and played for another couple of months. Mr. Kellogg was happy to continue playing my contract for the start of the new year, but he decided to stop his sports venture. He put my contract up for sale for 200 Million Dollars. He told me to wait at home until there is a new investor interested in my contract.

To finish with this playing run, I was called by Ms. Gloria Vanderbilt and she told me Mr. Kellogg is off the scene. Right to the end, the cheaters were stopped. One player that used an illegal racket in one of my final matches had to get reprimanded and our match canceled, the opponent was subsequently arrested. My sponsors hoped I could find a new investor for my contract. They also pointed out my playing stopped again even though I was a winning player. I was still the number 1 ranked player.

Chapter Ten
The End of The End

The end of the end for my pro tennis did take place in late 1999. This was months after I had donated my tennis rackets to charity, and started to just work on my Architect profession. I received a solitary phone call one afternoon from a previous sponsor.

The phone call came from the Sutton East Tennis Center and my old sponsor told me he had a new sponsor interested in investing in my pro tennis playing. He asked me to meet them at the Sutton East Tennis Center courts at a given date and time to give a demonstration of tennis playing ability for the new sponsor. The one big problem I had to explain was that I don't have my tennis rackets any more. The organizer of the meeting told me he would supply a tennis racket to play with.

As like previous chapters in my playing I re-entered the front door of the Sutton East Tennis Center right on time. No big changes were made to the tennis center's decor. The glass panels dividing the lobby from my tennis court were still there. My personal changing room and toilet were also still there. I was starting to feel the exhilaration of returning to play more pro tennis. I looked to my right side then fully turned to the manager's office room. I looked through the doorway into the room and saw there was one of my previous sponsors and the new prospective sponsor sitting there. My new sponsor's name was Mr. Donald Trump. This was years before Mr. Trump was the star of the tv show *The Apprentice* and later elected President of the United States of America. Mr. Trump wasn't someone new to me. In fact, I had already seen him before through pro tennis playing and my job working in an Architect office.

From that time in my history, I had most recently seen Mr. Trump in 1994 while working for an Architect named Sonny. Sonny was not only a Licensed Architect but was one of the sons of a successful real estate investment family. In the early 1990's Sonny's family had a big financial downfall in their real estate business. There was an economic depression in the Real Estate Industry and the overall US economy. That is the main reason I started working for Sonny was a result of his financial situation. He had to put more time into making money as an Architect to pay the bills. Real Estate alone was giving him a shortfall in his balance books. He was in charge of selling some of the multi-story apartment buildings their family owned to recover from personal bankruptcy. To achieve this some of Sonny's buildings were put on sale, and in the depths of the recession, Mr. Donald Trump was financially able to bail out Sonny's problems with the purchase of these apartment buildings. At that time, I was in Sonny's home-office in Long Beach, NY. late at night. There was a phone call and Sonny was talking on the telephone about these real estate transactions with Mr. Trump. The office telephone speaker system was turned on. After I was introduced to Mr. Trump in the room, the three of us could hear each other. The subject of the conversation quickly changed to Sonny helping me to get back on the tennis court and start playing more pro tennis.

My employer Sonny had no idea that I was a pro tennis player. I didn't tell him and always kept shut about my pro tennis playing. He didn't know the level of my tennis successes either. After I started to tell Sonny some details about my playing career he did however recognize my player name Carlos Scipio. He told me he used to see me playing pro tennis on television stations that were broadcast in the Philippines. He also said he used to see me answer questions in interviews on these broadcasts. Sonny told me about how he was playing his own game of club tennis locally in Long Beach, NY. I asked him if he wanted to hit the ball around on the tennis court but he declined. I was surprised and didn't know why. I didn't have to play an intense tennis match. I knew how to hit the ball around for family and fun tennis. I didn't tell him about pro tennis and sponsors making big money from my tennis playing. This might have become a change in history with a lot of money getting made from my pro tennis playing.

I don't really know if meeting Mr. Trump and Sonny in a telephone conversation was the reason that Mr. Trump considered me for sponsorship years later. Some years went by from the time Sonny was asked to help me continue my tennis playing at his home-office, to when I started playing pro tennis again with Ms. Leona Helmsley. I was used to keeping my pro tennis from leaking out and at the time of the discussion of my pro tennis playing with Sonny I didn't tell the story to anyone. At the time, I had a full time day job for another Architect's office and was moonlighting at Sonny's Architect office to get more experience and make extra money to pay the rent.

During these years, I was also checking back with the Mitsubishi sponsors in Japan. After that meeting, I didn't ask Mitsubishi to call Mr. Trump to help with the sponsorship. This could have again been another history changing event. I didn't tell Mitsubishi anything about the conversation that night.

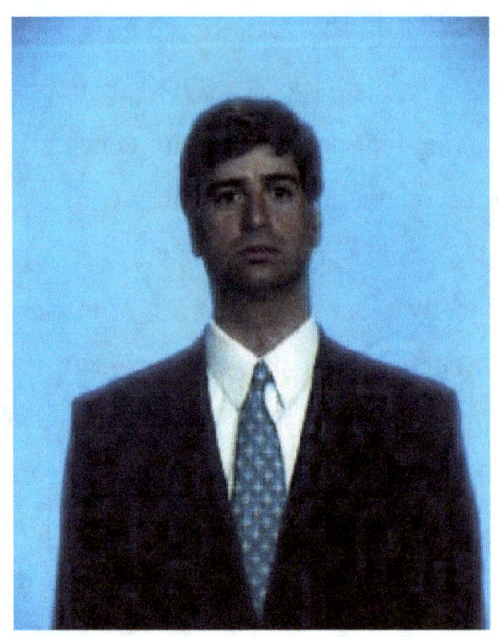

Photo: Portrait of John Riggio in 2001

As work mixed with my pro tennis on occasion, it was happening again at Sonny's office. I initiated to finish a supermarket and catering hall project that was sitting on his desk. The building's use was primarily for the Philippine community. A supermarket on the first floor and a Catering hall on the second floor. I made the whole project go ahead and after the completion of the construction in 1994 it culminated into a big opening day party event. Even Mr.

Donald Trump showed up at the ceremony. The event was productive for me and I met some important people from around the world along with making some new friends that were my own age.

The next week the Architect Sonny wanted me to marry Mimi. She was the daughter of a Pastor who led his own church in the Philippines. Sonny called her on the telephone first, then I was then given her phone number and we talked later at night. From our conversation we just talked about pro tennis. We stayed friends and she helped with my Hawaii visit in 1995.

Returning to the story in 1999 at the Sutton East Tennis Center, I talked to Mr. Trump for a few minutes. They paid the big ATP fees involved with this new tennis demonstration that was about to begin. I told Mr. Trump and the old sponsor that I no longer had my pro stock tennis racket and would need a new one. From the time I was young to the discussion with my prospective sponsor at 32 years old I still had never bought any tennis rackets myself. I was given all of my tennis rackets from Mr. Patrick Mulrooney of the S&S Sports shop or other by my new tennis racket brand sponsors. It would take until years later that I would start buying tennis rackets on my own.

The sponsors told me they would furnish me with new tennis rackets once the pro playing can start. The old sponsors handed me a used tennis racket that was laying around the tennis center. It was just an off-the-shelf racket and wasn't going to help my return to pro tennis playing. There was another pro player from the ATP on the courts. No match was to take place. I hit the ball well and was still able to move around the courts really well. Since the tennis racket wasn't of pro quality specification, it didn't make it through a full playing session. The racket frame bent and I just ended up returning it to the old sponsor when the playing was finished. He looked at the tennis racket and smiled knowing I still had the great strength to play pro tennis. I remember the bent racket just sitting on top of the desk in the manager's office.

The sponsors had me return to the lobby and chat for a while. They asked me about my ability to play pro tennis again and I said blankly that I would need a new pro stock tennis racket and maybe six months of playing to return to my previous sharpness. I might only need 2 weeks to play sharp, but the six-month time frame was too long for my prospective sponsors. The fact that I was even older at 32 years old was again the factor in the short wait time. This turned out to be my last time playing pro tennis.

I also started to shout out some of my problems from my side of the tennis center. One issue I explained is I was being left alone with my tennis career. I was no longer running my own tennis club and had problems finding tennis playing at a weekly pace. There were problems leaving my home environment behind and moving up to a stable pro life. I suggested some guidance on sports development and education. This was a similar request to when my coach in high school would give me definite names of books to read. Also, ideas of definite college education I could take. My sponsors understood the feedback I was giving them and they gave me a reply.

I did receive some phone calls months later but since there was no change in my training status. To search for tennis playing at that time was difficult. I was working full time and in off hours I would go to the weight gym. Unfortunately the new workout trend didn't provide an opening for tennis playing at these gyms. When I was younger I used to play on the courts alone to make my serves very accurate and my grips correct. The local courts had changed over the years. They now had a padlock and chains on them. I wasn't allowed to just walk on the courts anymore.

The stops in my playing made me think there was someone testing if I were a robot. A player that can turn on and turn off. After not playing tennis for one year. It obviously isn't possible to turn on like a robot and start playing sharp.

My new run at pro tennis playing didn't start again this time. There were too many weeks and months of wait time between regular tennis playing. I personally thought what was happening to the overall playing stoppages was absurd. I couldn't solve the playing problem myself.

As my workout returned home. I was jogging back at the track of my old high school in Jericho, NY. My regular six mile jog was consistent and kept me strong. One morning I was jogging on the track and noticed some school vehicles parked along the boundary of the public property. There they had uncovered some large trophies buried in the ground. A car drove near them and parked. I saw my old coach, Mr. Anthony Cambria, emerging from his automobile and walked over to the school workers excavating the trophies. He started to pick up the trophies and stock them in his car. These were some of the trophies he earned from my playing. They were also from other sports he administered at the school. When I was younger and winning tournaments Mr. Anthony Cambria had the trophies mailed to his office at the High School. The postal service and UPS would sometimes leave the boxes in front of his office door. From the delivery time to when Anthony picked up the boxes left room for the trophies to get lost. The morning haze was still burning off the grass as these lost trophies were recovered. It was a relieving feeling to see the trophies gleaming in the rising sunshine and making their way back to Mr. Cambria's office. Finally getting propped back up on a shelf to remember achievements of past tournament wins.

As I grew older, the pro tennis age limit for an adult player of 36 years old started to approach. Over that age you just become a senior tennis player and have no value. The simple hitting of the tennis ball with my racket was put at a stand still. It would take me a few years of waiting until I found a path to frequent tennis playing.

Chapter Eleven
Architect Career and Marriage

The transition from the bright lights of professional tennis to the world of architecture marked a significant pivot in my life—a shift that was filled with the promise of new beginnings and the pursuit of stability.

Ultimately, I graduated high school and as I continued to play professional tennis, I also made the definitive choice to pursue architecture. With a sense of purpose and focus, I enrolled in the New York Institute of Technology in the fall of 1997. My time at the university campus at Old Westbury, NY was rich with friendships and experiences, connecting with students who shared my ambitions while balancing my dedication to tennis whenever possible. I joined the student AIA (American Institute of Architects) chapter, actively involved in the school newspaper, and earned recognition through scholarships.

My new friends at college were involved with a fraternity Omega Delta Phi. They really took to my personality and were thrilled by my Pro tennis outside of school. I was made a star member of the fraternity, with a voting in ceremony, and remained in good standing through graduation.

The financial picture of my family was originally very healthy and stable but the end result was my only surviving parent was my Mother. She wasn't the one who knew how to run the income and payments. It was usually my father who had the financial knowhow and stability. These problems made it where I had to work a job to pay for most of my College expenses.

One job I earned was very solid and was arranged through my college's COOP program. I had to meet all kinds of requirements. This included having a high grade point average, references from my professors, and many interviews for my approval. I worked for the NYS Department of Education in their technical school district's Facilities office. The job was good. I worked fast and finished the big project they had me work on ahead of schedule. I was then distracted and took another job in the Architect field after that.

Most of the jobs after the COOP were 1099 freelance employment. This really meant I didn't have a job. It took years to figure that out. I was really working for myself.

This problem started to come through at tax time when I had to state my company name and deductions. This predicament was by mistake good training for self-employment. This is because after I received my Architect License I immediately started my own firm.

The people I worked for told me I should have a better job than what they had available. On one occasion, my coworker called someone they knew. The contact was an Architect with his own office. I talked to him on the telephone and he recommended I just work for whoever can hire me and just make my own office when I get older. This view of my work experience wasn't bad, but It didn't alleviate the problems they saw in my employment opportunities.

From the jobs I had, I started to put together a pattern of the work abilities employers needed me for. It was to make construction drawings for houses and buildings. This type of work is so hard and tedious and time-consuming that no one can do it correctly. It also involved reading the building and zoning code book. This involved memorizing many code requirements to build a new house or building. I did have the ability to do this kind of work.

The next ability that made my career become a reality was using the computer to make construction drawings. Computers were a new technology when I was young. Since I took the first classes they had available in computers, I was a pioneer in using Cad, computer-aided drawing.

In 1990 my college needed someone to draw the "Career Day" map on a computer. As I used to stop into their office to look for job listings. The Secretary asked me to make this drawing for them. It really came out great. I made one large print of the map and one small print. The small print was duplicated and handed out to the students in the college. To top it off I was paid for making the drawing.

My College schedule was very hard and I had to balance side jobs with College and Pro Tennis playing at the same time. I used to stay up all night long. Maybe I could get 1 or 2 hours of sleep at night. This usually happened at the end of each assignment and at quarterly tests in college.

My commitment paid off—by 1992, I graduated with the highest cumulative GPA for my Bachelor of Architecture degree. An accelerated 5 years degree, and accredited 1st professional degree. The Dean of the

Architecture College, Mr. Julio San Jose, personally awarded me the prestigious Gold Award for my accomplishments. My education and hard work led me to discover practical applications for my skills in the construction industry as I honed my craft.

Architecture offered a reliable pathway to financial stability. Instead of relying on an agent like many professional athletes, with the fluctuating payments from my tennis career, I found that working as an architect drew consistent income. This dual approach—pursuing architecture while engaging in sports—proved successful. I was able to pay my way through college, fund my own projects, and manage life beyond the drawing board.

My career path in architecture with NYIT was design and construction drawings. Seeing my drawings grow into built houses and commercial structures was my future. To many people, designing is very desirable and a lot of people want to do this.

My apprenticeship years were similar to my College years. The only difference is I was to accumulate 3 years' worth of work under a licensed Architect. As I worked I continued to gain work experience to make my future grow brighter.

A lot of my apprenticeship years were after my pro tennis contract was bought by Mitsubishi Japan. This was a time of tennis playing stoppage and phone calls off hours to Japan. Sometimes at work, I would talk about my pro tennis playing to my coworkers, all of a sudden they would turn into fans for a few minutes and ask me to sign my autograph. I was happy to oblige with my signature.

From 1992 to 2002, I worked a moonlight job for an Architect named Sonny in Long Beach, NY. I would drive 45 minutes at 10 pm to his office. It was an office in the converted 2 car garage of his house. There I would drop off CAD drafting work and pick up new work. It was on a 1099 but with my hustle, I made it as W2 as possible.

After I accomplished my apprenticeship work requirements, I only concentrated on obtaining my Architect License. This was coincidentally when my Pro Tennis playing started to pick up again with Ms. Leona Helmsley investing into my pro tennis contract. I was back playing at the Sutton East Tennis Center in Manhattan, NY.

This was a quiet time for my Architecture work. So I thought about the CAD software I used during College and my apprenticeship years and decided to make my own future and change to a different company. It was on the new

Windows operating system, and it really worked well on the new computer I just bought.

By March of 1998, I obtained my Architect License in the State of New York. This laid the foundations for the thrilling journey of entrepreneurship by establishing my own firm. From humble beginnings, I set up in a few empty rooms of my residence. I also adopted a shepherd dog named "Chopper".

There was a new future emerging. I would go to my job sites in the morning and make my construction drawings at night. I used the brand new technology of CAD drafting. I was still a pioneer and the first to make blue line drawings direct from my large print machine. This idea replaced old ammonium based blueprints made at a reprographics store. This was streamlining my work and saving me a lot of time. The building departments would look at my blueline prints and always said "this is the future of drawings".

From the time my elementary school suggested an Architecture profession to obtaining my Architect license and starting my own firm, I never talked about my father working as a Contractor. Most people would rant and rave about their father having his own contracting business. My father had his own construction company when he was young, at the age of 20 years old, and used to rebuild Brownstone apartments in Manhattan and Brooklyn, NY. After World War II he wasn't physically fit to work in construction anymore, but he was still able to buy a piece of property, hire an Architect, build a house and sell it. He used to tell me his secrets on how to develop a property and make a profit.

I was back advertising my architecture services. I used my computer knowledge to start my own website for my Architect Office called www.johnriggio.com. I have kept this url functioning ever since, and it helps to advertise my firm. Showing contact information, portfolio pictures and a description of my services.

My excellent work results for clients were starting to pay off. My business slowly started to grow. It took a few years but I expanded my business into a professional office space in Hicksville, New York. This move included my W2 employee, a drafter who helped me to make construction drawings for building projects. I also had consultants to expedite applications to the NYC Department of Buildings. My business was much higher than the offices I had previously worked for.

As I started to build my clientele, my day-to-day life morphed from playing pro tennis to navigating construction sites, meeting with clients, immersing myself in floor plans, and engaging in conversations about design with fellow industry professionals. The learning curve was steep, but perseverance was my ally. I experienced early successes and challenges, learning how to balance business logistics while also fostering creativity in my designs.

I also frequented visits to professional networking in Manhattan, NYC. Years earlier I regularly played pro tennis at the Sutton East Tennis Center in Manhattan, NYC. I knew how to navigate through Manhattan. The professional networking wasn't a singles night event. The networking was to take a break from working and get out to talk to like-minded people. It was with a good group of people. One was Mr. Justin Berber, an American music entertainer. Many networkers were part of big high-tech companies. Another co-networker I knew was Mr. Mark Zuckerberg who was just starting up Facebook. Others were lawyers helping entertainers and businesses. Some were involved with politics. Even the world richest were present and networking.

With Pro tennis and Architect work, I have known people in all of the different political parties in the USA; Conservative, Democrat, Republican, Freedom, Libertarian etc. This includes some US Presidents and some running for different political offices. One political party I met at professional networking was the Libertarian Party. They organized some networking events and we had dinner at a trendy restaurant together. One member was nice enough to propose making me a paid member of the party.

After the 9-11 attack happened in Manhattan, NY, during the year 2001, my social and business path changed from the center of the city to the perimeter areas. I was usually socializing and working between Long Island and the outer Boroughs in New York City at this time. In the midst of these horrible national problems there were still unexpected career progressions with my personal life taking an unexpected yet fulfilling turn. At one of the New York City permit offices, in Brooklyn, NY, I met a charming female expediter named Ms. Huijun (Anne) Wang, who was leaving her job as a permit expediter in training. She was interested in finding new opportunities in the world of architecture. This shared passion for architecture provided a solid foundation for our budding relationship.

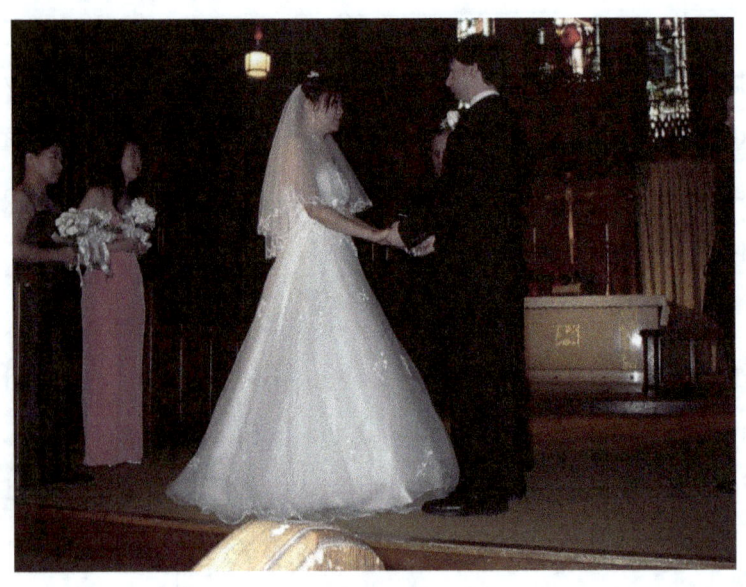

Photo: John and Anne's marriage 2004.

As our bond deepened, I invited Anne to join my firm, embracing the idea of building our professional lives simultaneously. With each passing day, our partnership blossomed into love, and soon we tied the knot, merging our professional and personal pursuits. Anne and I made the decision to relocate to Flushing, New York, intimately tying our growing family to the vibrant tapestry of the city. With my pet dog, Chopper, joining us, we found a new apartment, transforming our lives with shared warmth and laughter.

The atmosphere in Flushing, NY was mostly Chinatown. Huijun had arrived in the United States of America 6 years earlier from China. Learning the American English language was difficult and the neighborhood helped with this challenge. Joining the Christian church in the USA was a big change from having no religion. We frequented all of the local shops on Main Street, Flushing, NYC and it was a new experience for me.

However, the challenges of life did not cease with marriage. As my architectural practice broadened, I continued to relocate my office, eventually establishing a presence in Long Island City. There, I witnessed growth: moving to larger spaces to accommodate our expanding project load and distinct employee needs.

During this time, we welcomed our child, Nancy, she was very smart in school and we brought her to ballet lessons for many years. She performed in many dance shows going into her teen years. To accommodate our larger family we moved into a bigger apartment down the road in Elmhurst, NY. A place a lot like Flushing just with more shopping and a big Mall.

Even though our marriage agreement didn't allow previous siblings, Huijun's son Zhaowen from China came to live with us at the age of 12 years old. The whirlwind of family life intensified. My office continued to thrive, but I was always conscientious of balancing my work life with personal responsibilities. We used to go to church on the weekend and embraced new adventures together. This even included adopting a playful cat named Kitty for my daughter.

As with any journey, there were unexpected detours. The economic depression in 2008 sent ripples through the construction industry, challenging many architects, including me. As the demand for commercial projects dwindled, I adapted by refocusing my services on residential architecture. It required focusing my mind on creativity and peoples personal needs, but with determination, my team and I persevered.

Our family was starting to get on the move. Traveling to New Jersey on the weekends for shopping and children fun parks. With stops during the travel time, Nancy won first prize in a drawing competition at a Diner in Edison, NJ. We drove back to collect the gift.

Working in the Architect profession and the construction industry can keep you away from many distractions. This can have its good side and its bad side. When I was younger I used to run with the crowd, like going shopping at a new store or socializing at a popular establishment. Many times someone would spread the word among my friends to act timely on having fun or shopping and eating out. On the inside of architect and construction industry work, those types of group trends don't exist. You can however take on your own initiative and mold your own future. This is good but you have to watch for unknown circumstances. The Architect rules require continuing education. This is one thing every licensed Architect has to finish each year. This makes an Architect either study on the internet or go in person to an approved seminar event. This sole function keeps you up to date, but to expand your knowledge on business issues or other things, you will have to make your own way.

Growing from this kind of steady and monotonous lifestyle had brought about a slow move up and away from the original home town I lived in. The everyday getting up and going to work had brought a strange strength to keep the problems away. Having learned to keep a good alignment of work and home had made my new future good ahead with few obstacles.

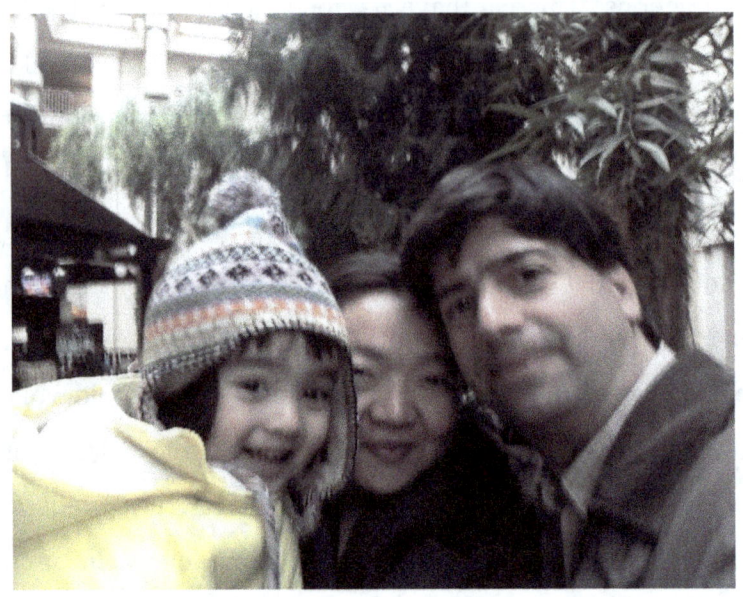

Photo: Nancy, Anne, and John in NYC 2007.

With the economic depression of 2008, everyone was starting to move out of town. I continued nurturing my architect firm, John Riggio, RA Architect, LLC, which expanded into Metuchen, New Jersey. This is a Borough in the middle of the Township of Edison, NJ. Many people were moving from our areas in New York City to these areas around Edison, NJ and Central New Jersey..

With our new life in New Jersey our daughter Nancy, grew strong in elementary school and showed incredible talent in basketball, making her a local star at a young age. She had crowds of people cheering for her in the gymnasium.

As the personal family life and architect business progressed. There was still an overboiling of events that came from living in New York City. The sailing away on architecture with my wife and family would come to a sudden halt.

There were problems developing in our family from interference following us from NYC and misguided directions on personal and business development. The culmination of these problems forced a simple divorce from my wife. This is a common occurrence in the USA, and playing the new divorced family life just started to take hold. The shock of this family divide was then followed by a new family tragedy.

My mother Rose, who helped find that Prince tennis racket when I was 9 years old, passed out at the wheel of her car and the subsequent result of the auto accident killed my oldest brother Paul. My mother never returned back to our family home and instead lived in a nursing home. Just a few years passed in the nursing home and Rose succumbed to old age and died in the hospital.

Rose's "Will" was settled a short time after her death. I remember my sponsors telling me there was a trend for groups of people from different countries like Puerto Rico that assist in stealing money from Pro tennis players. They are part of an elaborate plan of crime to infiltrate pro sports players families structure and then funnel money from the pro athletes' conservatoriums. They were also exploiting players not receiving money from the conservatoriums. These instabilities were real and the stories I was told are from years of experience of analyzing crimes against sport players.

Anne and I didn't go for new marriages and children like a lot of people do, instead we continued many of the same family functions together. One thing we still did together was go on vacations. We had some nice group tours together to places like; New Orleans, Miami, New England, etc. This worked out great and was a great success.

At home we kept our family responsibilities and Nancy earned a place in advanced highschool. As she attended the school, I was eager to help her success. I volunteered in the school's PTA and after some experience with them I was voted the PTA President. I initiated a new fund raising drive that in return gave donors a new T-shirt with the school's logo on it. Nancy is now thriving as a college student. My architectural firm and career has continued to grow. I find solace in what I have built—a career fueled by my childhood passion, a family enriched by memories, and a future filled with possibilities. In embracing change, facing challenges head-on, and nurturing creativity, I remain committed to moving forward in all aspects of life. This chapter serves as a reminder that every turn, whether in love or profession, has driven me closer to who I am today.

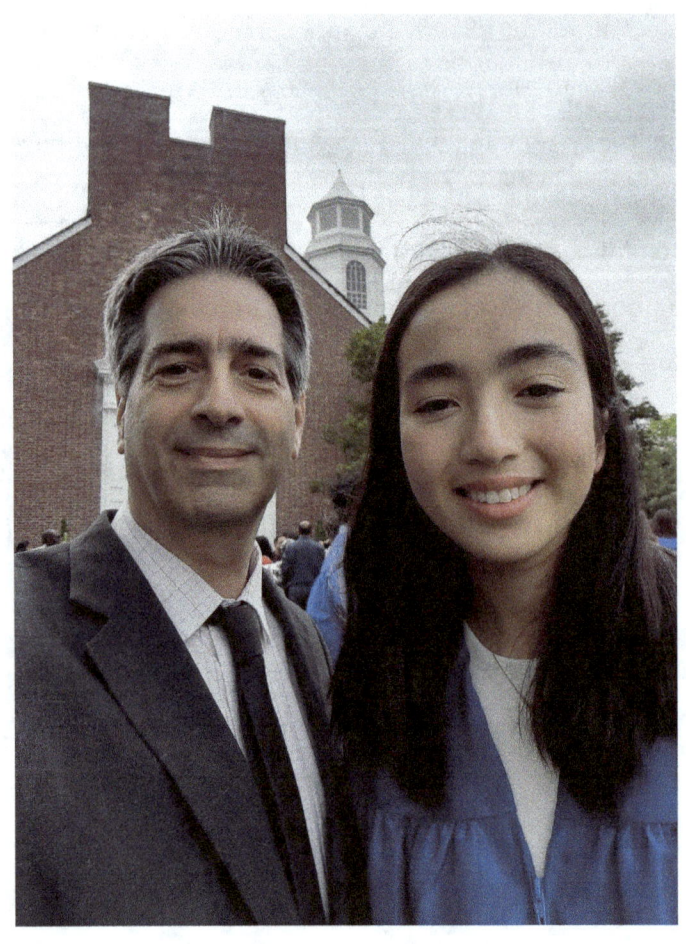

Photo: Nancy Riggio's High School graduation 2023.

The office in Metuchen, NJ has been the stage for my radio shows and video podcasts in the past years. Since the shows are centered on my Architect profession my office is the perfect place to take the spotlight. There had been a lot to talk about with my office growing slowly over the years and my project volume also increasing. recently averaging over 100 projects per year. There have been some ups and downs in the economy that made for a variation in the number of projects in other years. With my aptitude to work on construction projects, I have accumulated a long list of quality designs throughout the years.

Recently, I have been designing large one family houses. With a balance of commercial projects that include restaurants, etc. This is different from the past years of designing Gas stations with convenience stores and US Government recruiting offices. There were also a lot of medical offices and one / two family houses in previous years. The main goal of my Architect office is to provide an income to live on. Growing my business and my income are a top priority.

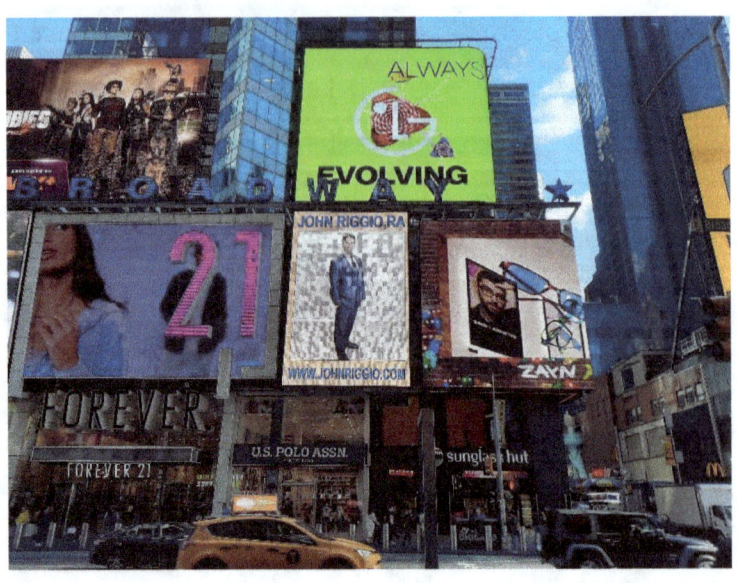

Photo: My billboard in Times Square, New York City 2022.

In an effort to build a smarter and better office was my new goal. I had gone through the great depression of 2008 and some other economic ups and downs. To start improving my office I started to take more educational classes in business. These basic classes were on the internet and I was able to take a few hours to study and make new improvements to my office functions. Also, the podcasts I have been making were having me reflect on my past years and help to improve my overall business picture. My efforts have succeeded and I now have employees working on a w-2 form. I even went through some office space expansions and improved the office decor with new business furniture. I further upgraded my computer systems and started to buy serious business computers and print machines for the office. This was also a big break for the influence of my employers of years past, who always bought cheap home computers to work on business CAD software. I once worked at an office where my desk was an old wood door layed on top of a file cabinet. These kinds of work examples weren't helping to influence my future.

Reflecting on my journey, I stand at the intersection of architecture and family, cherishing the lessons learned along the way. This chapter has taught me that life is rarely linear; it is woven with the threads of victory, setbacks, and resilience. Each experience, every relationship deepened along this journey, constructed the foundation for my personal and professional life.

Chapter Twelve
Returning To Tennis and Onward

As I navigated the waves of life after 1999, a significant chapter unfolded—a transition from the fast-paced courts of professional tennis to the more grounded yet equally challenging realm of architecture and family life. At the age of 32, with the flame of my professional tennis dreams flickering out, I found myself at a crossroads. The local tennis courts had locked their gates to me, and I began to feel the weight of uncertainty pressing down on my shoulders. I had not only turned away from the sport I once submitted but had also allowed the memories to fade like photographs left too long in the sun.

The decision to donate my tennis rackets to charity was both cathartic and somber. In relinquishing those instruments of my past triumphs, I thought I was closing a chapter. Yet, in the back of my mind lingered the echoes of applause, the scent of freshly mowed grass on a court, and the rush of adrenaline that came with a fierce rally. But life, as it so often does, swept me away on currents of responsibility. I began to forget, to sidestep the memories that once defined me, focusing instead on my architectural endeavors and raising a family.

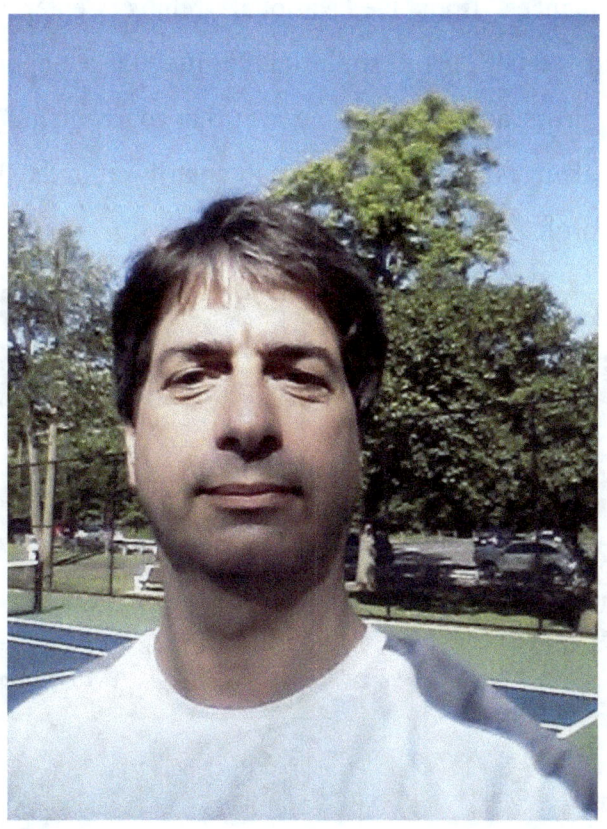

Photo: John Riggio on the tennis courts Edison, NJ in 2018.

Years passed, and my journey carried me through the bustling streets of Manhattan, where I delved into the world of professional networking. I mingled with industry leaders in High Tech, Finance, Politics, Business, and Professional careers engaging in conversations that sparked dreams and ambitions. Fate intervened one evening at one of these networking events, where I bumped into former acquaintances from the National Tennis Center. They greeted me with warm smiles and politely asked about my career years ago. "Didn't you win that tournament?" they asked, their words pulling me momentarily from the depths of my professional identity.

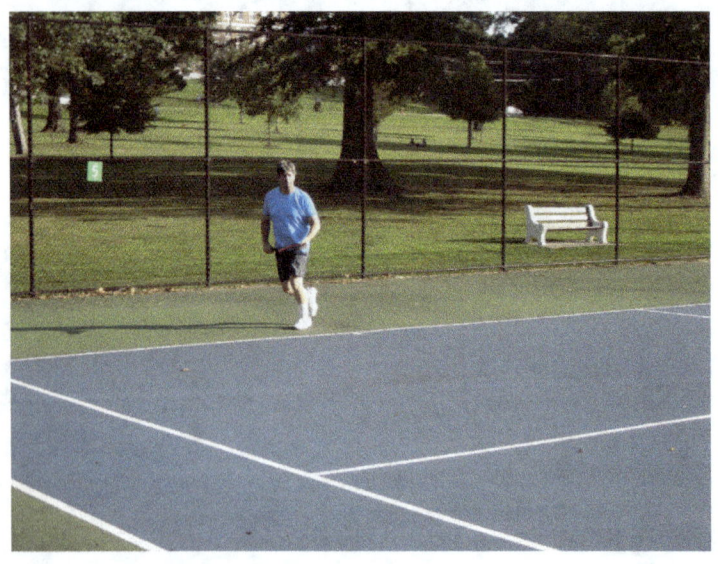

Photo: John Riggio on the tennis courts Edison, NJ in 2020

Though I recognized their faces, their inquiries were but fleeting whispers in the wind. I had let slip all those remarkable moments—the thrilling matches, the steely rivalry, the glory of defeating formidable opponents. I brushed aside their reminiscences as I focused on the discussions about building designs and blueprints. Tennis felt like a past life, relegated to distant memories, overshadowed by the responsibilities of adult life.

However, I would not remain in oblivion. It wasn't until nine years later, during a day spent with my daughter at Astoria Park, that I rediscovered the game that once filled my heart with joy. We strolled from the children's play area, and ventured closer to the running track. The thrill of something familiar tugged at my spirit as we passed by a couple of empty tennis courts. One was alive with activity, where a coach was giving lessons to a few eager students. Intrigued, I approached.

"Could you teach me tennis?" I asked, my heart racing like it had in years past.

"Absolutely!" he replied. "It will be $60 an hour."

A mixture of excitement and trepidation coursed through me. Was I really ready to plunge back into the world I had forgotten? I felt like a novice approaching a game I once mastered. "Great," I responded. "Let me buy a racket, and I'll be back next week."

The journey back to tennis began with a simple trip to the store. I purchased 3 starter rackets, the kind you could find on a shelf at a department store, and my daughter and I returned to the courts for our first lessons.

It was as if I were starting all over again. The sensation of holding a racket felt both thrilling and foreign, like stepping into an old pair of shoes that had grown stiff with neglect. I was utterly out of practice; my swings were awkward, my footwork cumbersome. With every strike, I was reminded of those carefree childhood days, yet I felt like a five-year-old, tentative and clumsy, grappling with the basics of the game. My daughter, too, was finding her path, absorbing the instruction with natural enthusiasm, and it sparked a flicker of pride in me.

Unfortunately, the years had been less than kind to my physical condition. Over the years, the stress of balancing work and family had manifested into a concerning weight gain—I had ballooned up, carrying an additional one hundred pounds. Reinventing my fitness regimen became essential. The lessons at Astoria Park not only served to jumpstart my tennis skills, but they also motivated me to confront my weight issues head-on. With a renewed focus on jogging and healthy eating, I gradually shed the layers of weight that had enveloped me.

Through perseverance, I improved my game steadily. The instructor encouraged me and even mentioned that he occasionally stopped by the National Tennis Center. Driven by curiosity and a desire to challenge myself further, I inquired about league play. I learned about Level 1 doubles matches. With an insatiable urge for competition rising within me, I signed up.

Returning to the National Tennis Center was surreal. I could hardly believe I was stepping back onto courts filled with the thrill of competition. My first matches were spirited yet humbling. The echoes of laughter and the shouts of athletes fueled a nostalgia I thought I had buried. I played doubles, rediscovering strategies and spins, and slowly began to regain my game. Although I was rusty, I found joy in the camaraderie that doubles play fostered. To my surprise, I managed to win the 2.0 doubles league 3 times by gaining the most points, and ultimately clinched a modest 2.0 doubles tournament title. With each win, I received a gift.

I was also slowly figuring out what tennis rackets to use. From the off the shelf tennis rackets at the department store to the integral frame rackets at the sporting goods store. The Prince Tennis racket started to re-emerge again when I bought the Prince gold racket. It was the start of some winning games, even a tournament, at such a low level. The progress with the rackets did help and I could feel it was also joined with better tennis playing.

However, it wasn't long before I noticed a paradox at the National Tennis Center in Flushing NY: the absence of singles matches. Out of sheer curiosity, I asked the staff at the front desk why singles games weren't available. Their response left me puzzled. "We just don't hold them," they said. I couldn't fathom why these exhilarating one-on-one matches were so hard to find. The pursuit of singles felt like an elusive dream, one I couldn't quite reach.

As I started to rekindle my thirst for the game, the memories of my younger years began to resurface, weaving together a nostalgic tapestry filled with recollections of my early triumphs and the sensations of competition. I searched the internet and found the Alley Pond Tennis Center had singles tennis and drills. I started playing tennis at Alley Pond, but had completely forgotten about my pro playing years ago. I brought my daughter to watch me play some matches and drills. She watched my matches through the windows at the tennis center. Although years had passed, when I began to play, I felt the flicker of muscle memory returning. I was determined to gradually reclaim my skills, steadily moving up through the ranks of Level 1, Level 2, and onto Level 3. Each session marked a new achievement—a celebration of the small victories that bred confidence and enthusiasm.

The journey continued as we relocated to New Jersey, where opportunities to encircle my daughter Nancy in the game burgeoned. I enrolled her in "Quick Start" tennis programs at Garden State Tennis—full of energy and excitement, she quickly adapted to the game, and I reveled in coaching her alongside her formal training.

Encouraged by my daughter's evolving knowledge to play tennis, I began to share stories of my past in the sport. I recalled tournament victories and cherished victories that shaped my character. Each memory painted vibrant images in both our minds—the electric atmosphere of the crowd, the pressure of championship matches, and the sweet taste of victory.

The rise of social media ushered in new avenues for connection that I had not embraced before. I joined Meetup.com and found myself embedded in various tennis groups throughout Central New Jersey and North New Jersey. My network blossomed; I explored leagues such as the USTA Flex League and some indoor club leagues at Chatham and Nassau Tennis. Again sharing laughter and camaraderie with fellow players. Despite my advancing age, I felt invigorated, buoyed by the life each match imbued within me. The flex league started to jolt my mind into remembering my pro tennis years. I was starting to remember bits and pieces of the past. I knew from my age and playing ability it was going to take a long time to play like my younger years.

My wife, Anne, only played a little amount of tennis. Winter was closing in and she needed to visit her family in China. We made travel plans to visit the city she grew up in named Karamay, China. This is located in the northwest part of China, called the Xinjiang Province. Their family was part of a contingency of government workers that originated in Beijing, China. They are living there primarily to develop the oil resources of the Province. She told me her first cousin was a top female tennis player from the province they lived in. For this trip to China, I brought my Babolat Aero Pro tennis racket. This was a sturdy tennis racket that was a revival of a teardrop shaped head. That was different from my precision shaped head tennis rackets of years ago. This racket helped my ball speed go up and made my tennis game play like I wasn't an embarrassment on the court anymore. Anne's cousin stayed involved with tennis after her glory years and was teaching tennis at the local courts. I was able to play some games of tennis with her and some of her students. It was a lot of fun. It was wintertime in China but the tennis playing didn't stop. We played outdoors and indoors.

When we returned to visit her cousin's parents' residence there was some quiet time to talk about tennis. I haven't been thinking about my pro tennis years. To my surprise, Anne's cousin walked into the room with my pro tennis player trading card. She was a big collector of tennis trading cards and was already a big fan of mine. She flashed me the card. She already knew I was the number 1 player. Years ago they used to watch me play tennis on cable television. She remembered me winning the world renowned American Airlines Tournament and the Manhattan Open along with the nice prize for the victory.

Back home, the fluctuating levels of engagement within the tennis community prompted me to take initiative. Eventually, I established my own Meetup group: the Central New Jersey Tennis Meetup. Fueled by my passion, the aim was to create an active community for players of all skill sets to come together. In June of 2016, the project launched, and with a blend of enthusiasm and diligence, I amassed a rotation of over 1,700 members—a diverse collective of adult males and females committed to nurturing a love for the game.

Through ups and downs, the foundation for the group solidified, even as external circumstances such as the COVID-19 pandemic posed challenges the group still grew. Many people wanted to play tennis outdoors in the fresh air at this time. The health benefits of playing tennis during COVID-19 were important to people in my group.

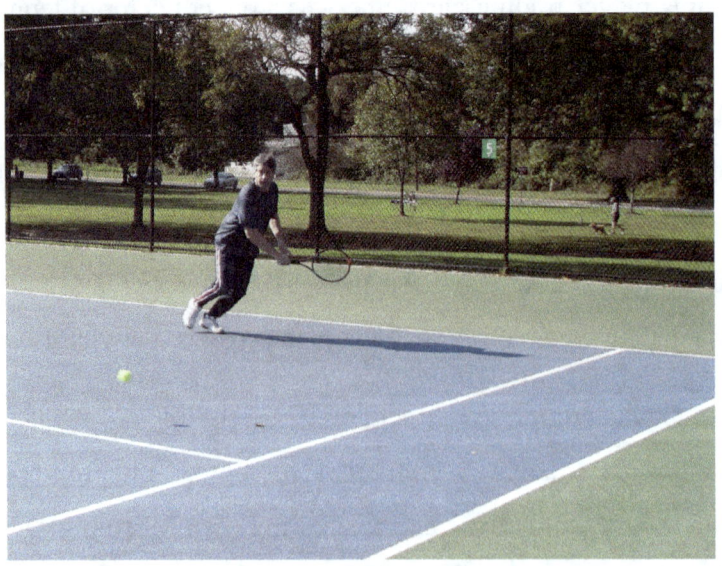

Photo: Playing tennis with my group.

I have one event each week that teaches tennis to a group of adult players. They usually have to go to the local department store and buy a tennis racket off the shelf for the first time. I teach them the basics; How to stretch their muscles to play tennis, how to hold the racket handle. The grips are Continental (Hammer), Eastern, Semi-western, and Western. I also go through the backhand grips with Continental (Hammer) and the Eastern backhand. I then show the group how to position themselves to hit the ball. Swinging from the shoulder. The next important skill is to hit the ball in front of your body. I like to tell them to hit the ball like a "fly swatter". I then instruct them how to stand at the baseline located at the centerline of the court. Remembering to hold the racket in position using two hands and bending your knees. All of these things lead to more and more lessons of hitting the ball forehand and backhand, net play, and serving. The students learn very quickly and like returning for additional lessons.

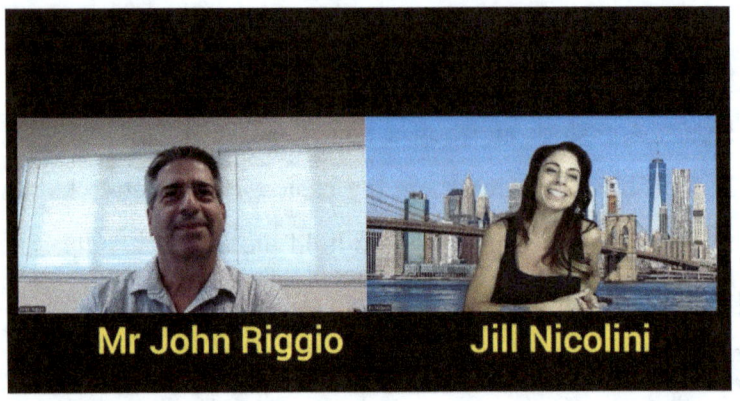

Photo: Podcast Business News show with host Jill Nicolini.

After returning to playing tennis I realized that the safety of getting nurtured from a young age to play tennis and learn tennis at a decent pace wasn't there anymore. Splashing back into tennis at the age of 39 was difficult. Even though the tennis was just low level recreational tennis the direction back was very slow and involved hopping around to different tennis centers and trying out different kinds of learning. There were group tennis drills that taught people how to approach a ball and hit it across the court. Other Tennis was double or single tennis usually on a weekday night. This is when everyone was finished with work and played for a couple of hours. As I started playing with my own tennis group I have found my mind to slowly remember tennis. Teaching the fundamentals of tennis to adults, who just picked up the tennis racket for the first time, has made my game have more foundation on it. I noticed that I had to start, stop and then start again after remembering my tennis playing from a young child.

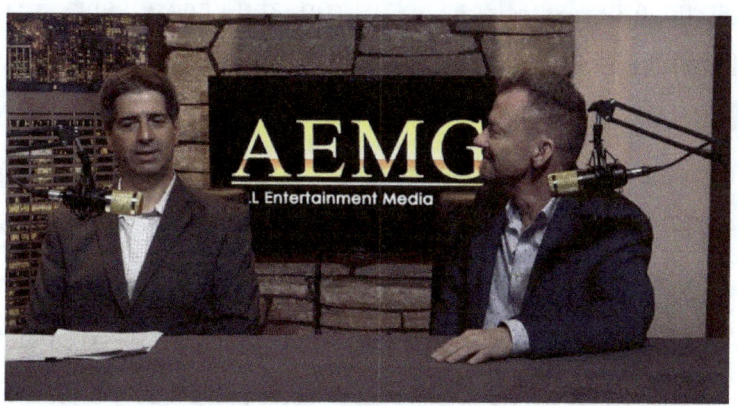

Photo: In-studio PBN show with host Mr. Steve Harper.

From years of breaking tennis rackets when I was younger, my return to tennis at 39 years old produced no broken rackets. I have however started to accumulate all of the old tennis rackets from the past. I bought the pair of Ms. Evonne Goolagong and the Mr. Marty Riessen tennis rackets my parents had from years ago and all of the old wood tennis rackets we had in the house. The old tennis rackets from my preteen years and high school years I have also searched for and purchased. I finally figured out how to find some of my old pro stock tennis rackets and now own a few of those too. There are still more rackets to buy.

In recent years, I found a different way to showcase my journey and expertise through broadcasting. Engaging with Business Talk Radio about my Architect professional career in the New Jersey, New York and Pennsylvania area. This nationally broadcast radio program to help discuss my professional work and help advertise my Architect office also started to revive memories of my pro tennis playing career. One of the Business Talk Radio shows I was answering a question of how I decided to work as an Architect? I started to explain about shifting to Architect work because it was proven to work alongside pro tennis players. I widened the details of my answer with naming tennis players I knew in the past and some names of tennis tournaments. This opened new doors to share not only my architectural passions but also the stories from my earlier proficiency in tennis—an overlap of my two passions. This series of nationally broadcast Business Talk Radio shows with host Ms. Jill Nicolini, went on for more than a year.

As I transitioned into the video podcast format with the Podcast Business News, I started talking about my tennis career from years past. As I talked about these old stories some interest grew. The reflections triggered a resurgence of memories surrounding my matches and tournaments. As my memories started to grow again I started documenting my journey in writing. Years ago I didn't write anything down. I was told times, dates, locations, with facts, and figures just verbally communicated. Every episode became a tapestry, interweaving themes of perseverance, laughter, struggle, and triumph. There was an in-studio show where I traveled to the Podcast Business News broadcast studio location by hired car and made 2 shows with the host Mr. Steve Harper. Half of the allowed show time was for my Pro Tennis stories and the other half was for my Architect career.

I created a website dedicated to documenting my professional tennis career, an archive comprising historical details of my career woven alongside proud reminiscences. Through diligent efforts, I chronicled my astonishing record: a decorated career that encompassed about 155 tournament wins. Approximately 40 as a junior and 115 as an adult player. Along with that webpage I have introduced a Facebook.com page titled "John Riggio Pro Tennis Player". The page has many photographs and video clips from the years gone by.

Moreover, the legacy of my time with sponsors like Mitsubishi remains embedded in this tapestry. Although their lead in my contract ultimately came to an end, I still had an open invitation to visit Japan. I started trying to remember the names and telephone numbers from long ago. It took months to find my sponsors in Japan. I used the internet and was finally able to locate some information. I first visited on a tour with my daughter Nancy. The tour was run through a company from Japan. It had a theme of religious and civic buildings. I even made a podcast on Podcast Business News from my hotel lobby in Japan with the host Ms. Jill Nicolini, describing what I saw about Tennis and Architecture. I had to make the time within business hours here in the Eastern United States and not too late in Japan, where I was staying. The hotel was very expensive and had a very nice waterfall in the background. This was a good preliminary trip. As I arrived in Japan and started traveling with the tour group, It was good to realize that Japan was a lot like the USA in many ways. One was shopping at the convenience stores like I do back at home. The familiar stores and ability to travel around each city, helped to forward a better search for my sponsors.

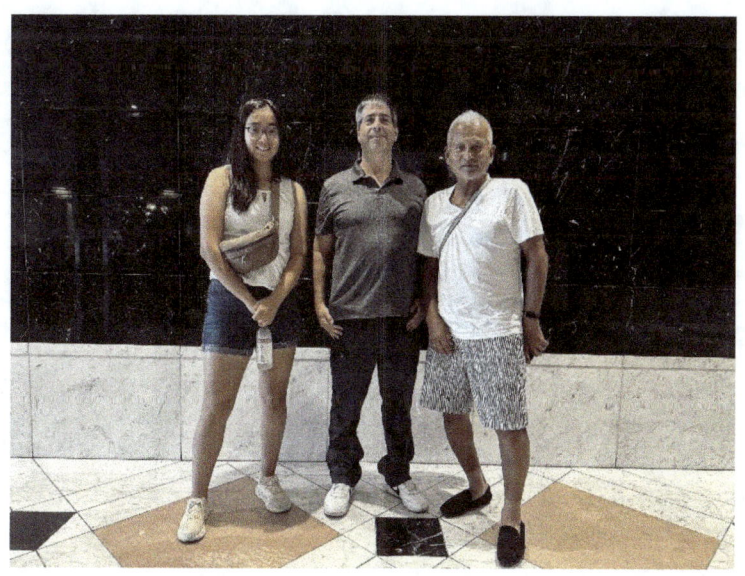

Photo: Nancy Riggio, John Riggio, Shigeyuki Nishio, 2024

The next year, I searched harder and located definite names and numbers. The new tour was reserved and, with Nancy coming along for another vacation, we traveled to Japan. The tour reserved a stay at the Keio Plaza Hotel, Tokyo, Japan. It was a very nice high-rise building complex with two towers. The weather that week was hot and in the 90 degree range with clear skies. On a Sunday, I was fortunate enough to finally rekindle ties with Mr. Shigeyuki Nishio who had once championed my career. We talked and caught up on old times. Mr. Nishio is still teaching tennis in Japan and is involved with the sport. The high times of pro tennis are past but the sportsmanship of tennis playing continues. Those connections felt enriching—full of nostalgia—reminding me that each step taken in the game had shaped my identity in tennis.

The journey has come full circle, allowing me to embody the spirit of both an architect and a player—not only redefining what success looks like in each journey but also ensuring that I pass down invaluable life lessons to my daughter, Nancy. As I pen this chapter, I feel anchored in purpose; these reflections guide me as I look forward to new horizons.

My story, one intertwined with tennis and architecture, continues to find new expressions. Each swing, each lesson, and every moment shared on and off the court have contributed to the multifaceted life I now lead. Rediscovering tennis has reinvigorated my passion, inspiring creativity that flows back into my architectural practice. The chapters ahead are not solely mine to write; they belong to my family, the community I've built, and the passion I impart to the next generation. Victory lives on in every heart I touch, whether it be through the elegance of tennis or the artistry in architecture. Indeed, the lines of the court and the lines of a blueprint are not so different—they both represent the boundaries of a world waiting to be forged by dreamers and doers alike.

As I move forward, my experiences with deceit in tennis became the foundation for my own personal resolve: to fight against these injustices, to support clean play, and to mentor the young talents who hoped to navigate a world often tempted by shortcuts. Ultimately, I chose to live by the adage my father imparted, steering clear of the shadows of dishonesty in a world that desperately needed the light of truth.

In the present, my efforts to sustain my pro tennis career continue unabated. My trips to Japan to meet sponsors, and efforts to generate content through videos and podcasts, place me in a never-ending quest to combine my love for the sport of tennis and the entertainment world that surrounds it. My journey is a testament to the resilience required to thrive, both as an athlete and as an individual in the face of challenges that constantly redefine success.

Chapter Thirteen
In Conclusion

The story continues about Mr. John Anthony Riggio, an American pro tennis player's life. As you have read up to now, there have been a lot of steady advances in my playing tennis career. My tournament wins and my contract prices rose to historic levels. My legacy as a player was also setting new records in ATP professional tennis. This pro tennis story started from a young age to my thirties and beyond. Me and my sponsors and coaches always played an honest game and stopped any cheating in our path. This gave us many years of success in pro sports.

My story overall has a typical set of circumstances for a pro sports player. The pro sports life and everyday home life. As I have described, home life takes on its own world. Usually a job to pay for everyday expenses and this acts as insurance so you don't fall too low. Whenever there was a play stoppage, I always stayed calm and used my own knowledge to keep my pro playing going. The confidence I had in my tennis playing made me search for more help.

Sometimes my search involved risking high level phone calls to stimulate my pro playing to continue on.

In the times I was waiting at home my sponsors would send someone to check on my well-being. Some interested people would just drive up to my family's home and talk for a while. The conversations were usually about my upcoming tennis matches and a quick look at my neighborhood. They also hoped I was getting all of my pro sports perks. Some of these things were owning a nice sports car. More importantly a nice girlfriend and potential wife to support my pro career.

In younger years, some interested tennis people would watch from far away at my home activities. Some of them watched my athletic involvement in sports with my home friends. They would tell me later that they could see I was a stand out playing those neighborhood games.

The personal relationships I have experienced are stated in this book to give you an idea of the entertainment world and the home world. The striving to succeed in sports and entertainment was intense. It was fast paced at many times with quick decisions on getting married and sharing in work and life.

When the pro tennis playing was over my Architect career made it where I could still strive at work and life. I didn't have to fall too low. The pro tennis world was a secret and I wasn't bragging about my winnings at home or at work. The hard work it takes to achieve your goals at anything was very real. I have explained about knowing some successful people you see on the news on television each night. The hard work never stops. From early morning to late at night. I was typical of any American kid having a limited number of options to take. Really concentrating hard on achieving in each direction I took was very important. Working long days and nights were necessary to achieve.

I have just shouted out loud many pieces of my history in this book. I have been telling you all of the details, names and places, but in the past, I didn't tell anyone! Sometimes I forget myself. If a stranger would ask out of the blue "Are you a pro athlete?" I would say "No". I was excellent at keeping my pro tennis and other experiences top secret.

The pro sponsor's game was to keep advertising and promotion away from my personal life most of the time. This was to keep me playing at my best. The camera boom from the TV truck that might turn on or might not turn on. There was no way I could tell. All of these things are made so I wouldn't get distracted. This developed to having a stand-in and spokesman travel and take interviews for my pro sport playing. From these experiences I have described there are many of my fans around the world and they have my playing cards.

The requirements the ATP had of having an alias name when playing a pro tennis match became frustrating. The original idea to have a player name was in good faith to protect my personal life, this includes my family and finances. This was a good idea in theory to have a safe home life and then run wild with a stage name and really make a big show. Unfortunately, this idea was easily infiltrated. Maybe years earlier or even generations earlier this idea worked for pro sports players, but the organized crime people are more sophisticated now. They can find you and your family very easily. There wasn't a definite way to stop these problems.

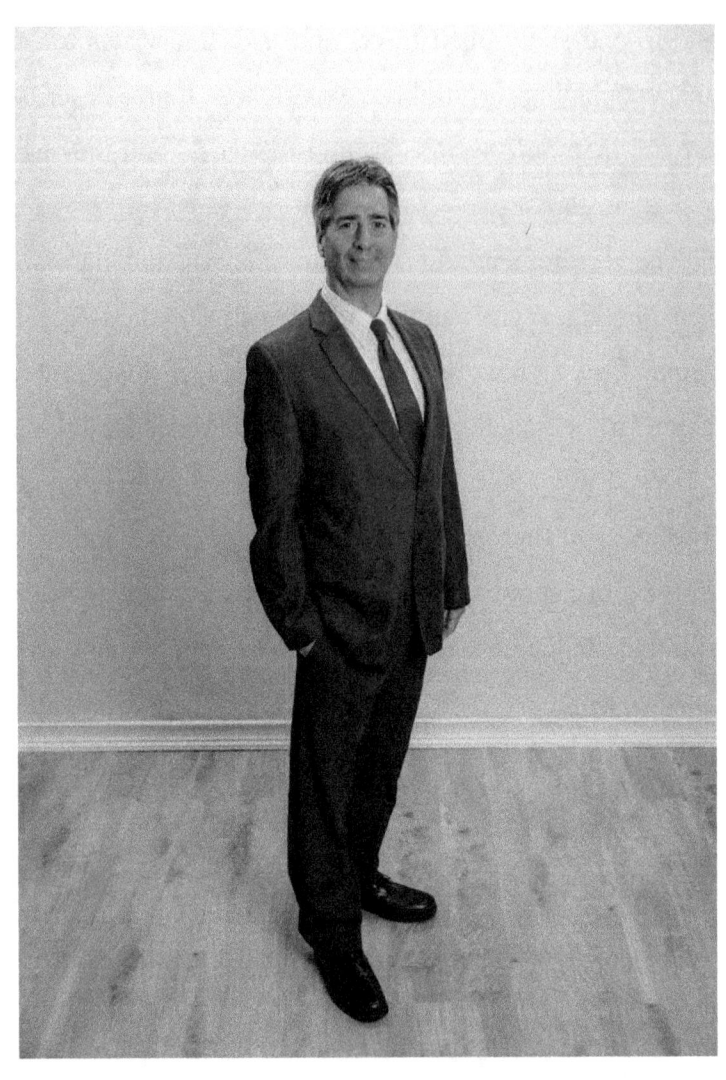

Photo: John Anthony Riggio in 2022.

Changing my player name with each contract investment started to build up anxiety on me and my supporters. As the years passed the idea of using my natural name John Riggio for all of my things was the best idea.

After reading this book you will have become very enriched by knowing about my tennis story and other players' tennis stories in the past. The people and players names I have listed might have been missed in your recollection of the sport. This book gives you the full picture of pro tennis and the correct one. Since I had the biggest tennis contract in sports history as a direct result of playing in the best tennis tournaments, that were authentic and well known around the world.

The tennis facilities I had were the best for real pro tennis playing. Not only that but the tennis facilities were based on a current trend that was designed by a higher authority presenting a contemporary feeling. The experiences of fans, television and sponsors watching were all there. I have mentioned a number of times the effort to improve my tennis center's ability to convey the tennis excitement and bring it to the fans. The tennis centers I had provided for frequent tennis matches, for the real-world of pro tennis, with basic accommodations for sponsors, spectators, lockers, rest rooms, etc. The most important part of my tennis playing centers were television broadcasts. This was what tennis was all about to me. I used to watch tennis on television at home on Saturday mornings. The matches could have been broadcast from anywhere in the world. I have found this was the real truth for my tournament matches. I have met people locally and from different parts of the world and they were able to confirm they saw me playing tennis and winning tournaments. They also saw me answering questions from sports news interviews on television. Cable television stations were the most far reaching with my matches getting shown on ESPN and other sports networks. Watching the best television stations give you the best tennis players.

I have spoken a lot about my professional career as an Architect. The main reason is my resurgence in telling my tennis stories has come through my Architect career. The audio shows I first made about my Architect career involved asking me questions about why I started working as an Architect. I honestly had to reply that my Pro tennis playing was an important part of why I am working as an Architect. From this answer, there was not only growing interest in my Architect work but also in my Tennis stories. The audio shows were gradually transformed into video shows on a podcast. On these new shows I continued to expand on remembering years past stories. This expansion of my tennis stories through my parallel life as an Architect is truthful.

As I share my stories with you in this book, I hope you can enjoy all of the excitement of the pro tennis years. This is because I was always an honest tennis player and had a great number of documented and solid state tournament wins and ATP pro tennis records.

I am still playing tennis on a regular basis with my Meetup.com group. This group I originally started in the spring of 2016 is like starting my tennis club in middle school all over again. It is the best way to play tennis and I am using my years of experience to run the games. The simple hitting of the tennis ball on the courts has kept me fine tuning my game. It has been ever so slow to progress back and play with a pro stock racket. The club has many playing members and is growing. There are many different people and levels of tennis getting played.

In my current chapter in tennis and in life, I don't have to wait for my sponsors to do anything. I have been taking a few minutes each day to compile my pro tennis history for every sports lover's curiosity and pleasure. The search for my tennis history has led me all the way to Japan and with great success. Sharing my memories of my tennis seen around the world wide has had a great impact.

I hope you can stay connected with my pro tennis playing career and life stories. Follow my video shows and internet articles to get more information about my playing career. There were so many stories packed into each year of my tennis playing that I can't fit them all into this book. I have told you the tale of my pro tennis origins and how it has led to my official title of a "Tennis Legend".

Tennis Tournament Levels

1. **American Airlines, Manhattan Open, Eastern Tournament, London Queens, Paris-Bercy, Lisbon, Portugal, Roland Garros**

    Other ATP tournaments: **Chicago, Illinois, Nashville, Tennessee, Dallas, Texas, Miami, Florida**

2. **US Open, Laver Cup, French Open, Wimbledon**
    Other ATP tournaments: **ABN**
    ATP Starter tournaments - **Vienne**

3. **Davis Cup, National Tournament (Pro tracks)**
    Other tournaments:

4. **ITF League tournaments - Minor Leagues**

5. **Level 5.5 and above playing**

    National Tournament (Amateur tracks), **US Olympic Team.**
    College Tennis (different tracks)

Note: The playing levels for Junior Tennis (under 18 years old) are the same as shown above.

Professional Tennis Player
Mr. John Riggio

Official "Tennis Legend"

Tennis Alias Names: John Strong, Carlos Scipio, John Vice, John Vanderbilt, John Rigo, John Holton, John Beast, Amadeus, Jack Racet

Nickname: "The Beast" or "The Beast Man" or "John Beast" (during Prince years.)

Full name: Mr. John Anthony Riggio

Country: United States of America

Residence: Rahway, NJ

Married Status: Ms. Dahlia - Engaged years 1981 to 1996 Ms. Huijun (Anne) Wang - Married in 2002, Divorced in 2014.

Spouse: Ms. Nancy Xuwen Riggio

Born: September 26, 1968, Roslyn, NY Long Island

Height: 5-11

Playing Weight: 155lbs

Plays: Right-handed forehand, One and Two-handed Backhand, Very fast ball speed.

Tennis Rackets: Babolat Precision Pro Stock Tennis Racket string tension 62 lbs.

Sponsored: 1977 S&S Proshop, Hicksville, NY.
1984 Prince Racket Company
1988 Slazenger Racquets.
1998 Dunlop Sports.

Pro Playing ended: 1999

College: Clemson University, Clemson, S.C. Supported Pro Tennis (only), from 1986

New York Institute of Technology, BArch 1992

Last Player Contract buyer price: $100,000,000.00 This was an ATP world record in 1991 for the highest price.

Last Player Contract Value: $150,000,000.00 dollars Plus

Last Player Contract offered price: $200,000,000.00

Highest Rankings, Men's Singles: 1 (one)

Ranking list,
ATP Men's Singles: 1500, 500, 200, 100, 26, 17, 9, 4, 1.

ATP Junior Men's Singles (under 18 years old): Ranked 1 in 1984-1985.

Winning Percentage: 24 out of 25, or 96%

ATP tournament wins: 155- Junior 40 and Adult 115 wins

ATP Tennis Records: Some ATP records set.
1.All-time record for the most ATP match wins in one season 1989.
2. All-time record for winning the most ATP first serve games in one season 1986.
3. All-time record for the highest percentage of last match in tournament wins 1985.
4. All-time record for the highest percentage of Tie breaker wins (100%) in one season 1985.
5. All-time record for the highest percentage game wins after I go ahead in the score of a match.1986
6. Highest percentage of comeback wins. This is when I lose the first match then win the remaining matches. 1986.

ATP Awards:
Won ATP award for the Junior MVP, Most Valuable Player of the Year in 1984.
Won ATP award for most winning Player of the Year in 1989.
Won ATP award for the Player of the Year in 1991.

Tennis Highlight: Scored the number 1 position in the world for Top Pro Tennis Fitness Test. 1985 to 1999.

Administrative Coaches: Mr. Anthony Cambria, Mr. Tony Scolnick, and others.